The
BOY
in the
SUIT

JAMES FOX

SCHOLASTIC

To the interlopers.
And to my family.

Published in the UK by Scholastic, 2024
1 London Bridge, London, SE1 9BG
Scholastic Ireland, 89E Lagan Road,
Dublin Industrial Estate, Glasnevin, Dublin, D11 HP5F

SCHOLASTIC and associated logos are trademarks and/or
registered trademarks of Scholastic Inc.

Text © James Fox, 2024
Illustrations by Tika and Tata Bobokhidze © Scholastic, 2024

The right of James Fox to be identified as the author of this work has been
asserted by them under the Copyright, Designs and Patents Act 1988.

ISBN 978 0702 33310 1

A CIP catalogue record for this book
is available from the British Library.

Printed and bound in Great Britain by Clays Ltd, Elcograf S.p.A.
Paper made from wood grown in sustainable forests and other controlled sources.

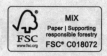

MIX
Paper | Supporting
responsible forestry
FSC® C018072
FSC
www.fsc.org

3 5 7 9 10 8 6 4

www.scholastic.co.uk

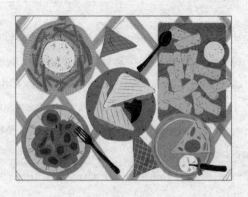

CHAPTER 1

Another day, another party in a grotty pub function room. I'd started to get used to going to so many parties. The chatting, the music, the getting nice and clean, and dressing up smart in my suit. I was becoming a proper party person.

Even after so much practice, I still got a weird feeling in the pit of my stomach just before I went inside. It was a sickly mixture of excitement and nerves, but mostly it was because I was hungry. Luckily, there's always food at parties.

"Look at me," Morag said as we approached the door. We stopped and she straightened my collar and adjusted my tie. "There we go. Looking nice and respectful. Nobody will suspect a thing."

I screwed up my face in anticipation. Usually Morag found some grubby stain or mark somewhere and tried to rub it away with her fingertips. But this time there was no stain because I had been sure to wash my face thoroughly. I braced myself for Morag's usual pre-party pep talk.

"So," she said, peering in through the steamy window, "it doesn't seem like anything out of the ordinary. Buffet to the left, bar to the right. Seating area in the middle. That's where we'll meet if anything goes wrong – got it?"

"Got it." I nodded like a soldier receiving orders. Morag's my mum, so I had to do everything she said, apparently.

A small group of partygoers appeared behind us, so we stepped off the path to let them through. My feet squelched in the mud. They nodded at us politely but didn't say anything.

"How do I look?" Morag asked.

"You look really nice," I said. "Like always."

Morag was wearing her favourite party outfit: a black leather jacket, black hat with lace that partially covered her eyes, smart black skirt with black tights, and black boots that came up to her knees.

"Thanks," she said, patting herself down nervously.

"Same procedure as usual. Quick in-and-out job – no drawing any attention to ourselves. Remind me what you're not going to do?"

"I'm not going to talk to strangers," I droned robotically. "Unless they talk to me first."

"Good. Anything else?"

I rolled my eyes. "I'm not going to have too much fun or make a scene."

One time I got too enthusiastic with the chocolate fountain and Morag would never let me live it down. She said it made us look *suspicious* and *not sad enough*. We couldn't go back to that particular church hall for a few weeks afterwards because they might have recognized us.

"And what will you do if anyone starts to ask you tricky questions?" said Morag.

"Go and find you," I recited. "In the seating area."

"Great, sounds like we have a plan." Morag began to walk towards the door. "Oh, I nearly forgot. We'd better check the name before we go in."

A sign had been placed on a wooden easel outside the entrance. It featured a black-and-white photograph of a smiling old lady with a cloud of wispy white hair on her head. She was surrounded by delicate illustrations of flowers, bumblebees and butterflies.

In Loving Memory of Ursula Grimsworth
1927–2023

"Poor sweetheart," Morag tutted. "Wasn't far off a hundred, bless her. Could've had a letter from the king."

This bit always made me feel weird, but we had to check whose funeral it was in case anyone sussed us out and asked us what we were doing there. That was the scariest part about not being invited, the risk of getting caught.

"Still," said Morag, "ninety-six – not a bad innings. Have you got the bags?"

I patted my pockets, and the plastic food bags rustled inside.

"Magic." Morag pushed open the heavy wooden door. "After you, Solo."

It wasn't the best funeral buffet we'd been to. The mini quiches were all cold and wobbly and white – I'm not sure they'd even been cooked properly. But it's like Morag always said: free food is free food, and beggars absolutely can't be choosers.

Morag was always going on about stuff like that. She reckoned there were people all over the world who would be grateful for a nibble at my leftover crumbs.

I poked at one of the squidgy quiches on the buffet table with my finger, trying not to throw up at the thought of the egg mashing between my teeth. It looked like cold, eggy sick served in a pastry cup. Quiche of any size, in fact, sat right at the top of my Official Top Five Worst Funeral Foods Ever list:

1. Quiche of any size, as I've mentioned. It looks, smells, tastes and feels like puke. There's *nothing* nice about quiche.
2. Olives. The sneakiest funeral food of all. They pretend to be innocent grapes, then ambush you with a mouthful of bitter grossness. Stuff can be hidden inside them too, like raw garlic and chilli. Horrible little secrets that only make them worse. Come to think of it, olives reminded me a bit of my dad, Jason.
3. Salmon and cream cheese on tiny crackers. These are at every wake without fail. It's not the taste that I hate, more the mess they made in my pockets when we tried to sneak them home.
4. Carrot sticks and that boring beige dip. Need I say more?

5. Oysters. You only find these at posh
   funerals, the ones with horses and carts that
   bring the coffin to the church. Morag once
   gave me an oyster and it tasted like slimy
   seawater mixed with snot. All the grown-
   ups were guzzling them as if they were
   delicious, like chocolate or pizza. I think
   Morag only pretended to enjoy the oysters.
   She always made a face when she has them,
   just like me.

"Either take that quiche or leave it, but don't *play* with
it, for heaven's sake," I heard somebody hiss like an
irritated alley cat.

My eyes jolted up to see an old lady waiting beside
me at the buffet, her empty plate in hand. She was
dressed in black from head to toe, with spectacles as
thick as window glass. Her hair was curled into tight
grey snail shells.

"Sorry." I quickly dropped the mini quiche on to my
plate, even though it made me want to gag. "I wasn't
sure I fancied it. Quiche makes me feel a bit… *sick*."

The old lady tutted and shook her head. Old people
were always mean, especially at funerals.

I shuffled down the table, investigating which of

my funeral favourites were waiting to be scoffed. I clocked all the usual suspects: sausage rolls, pizza slices, even sushi. Then I saw it. An untouched Mount Everest-sized pile of golden-brown breaded mozzarella dippers. Beside it, a glistening lake of sweet chilli sauce.

Here's the thing: breaded mozzarella dippers *always* get eaten first at funeral buffets. It's because they're factually proven as the best food ever. Plus everyone's sad, so they get really hungry.

I approached the breaded mozzarella dippers carefully, with a plan: I skip all the other foods and try to fit as many dippers as possible on to my plate, forming a foundation. Then I circle the buffet again, covering the first layer with stuff like pizza. Finally, I add another layer of dippers, which everyone else thinks is my first helping. I think it's kind of smart.

As I picked up the first mozzarella dipper with the metal tongs, the old lady shuffled next to me again, and sighed. *Abort Mission Dipper. Abort.*

"I can't say I have much of an appetite," she croaked. "It's just such a *sad* occasion. It feels wrong to be eating a finger buffet like we're at a birthday party."

I didn't know what she was going on about. There's *always* food at funerals – that's the whole point.

"Well, you should try to eat something," I said. "It's what Mrs Grimsworth would have wanted."

The lady smiled weakly and plopped a lonely cocktail sausage on to her paper plate. "Yes, yes, you're right. Ursula was always a generous host. Why stop now? Her platters of club sandwiches were so tall they would almost scrape the ceiling when she brought them through to the sitting room!"

"Sounds nice." I grinned. "I love sandwiches."

"Just because she's –" the lady paused – "*dead*, I don't suppose today has to be any exception."

"Exactly. Someone's paid good money for this buffet," I said, parroting Morag. "You might as well fill up while you're here. Make the most of it." I piled more mozzarella dippers on to my plate.

The old lady let out a small, sad laugh. "Well, it cheers my spirits to see a lad with such a healthy appetite." Her voice sounded faraway and wispy. "You remind me of my boys when they were small. Oh, how time flies." She took a crinkled tissue out of the end of her sleeve and started dabbing around her eyes.

"I'm having a growth spurt," I replied. "That's what everyone says, anyway."

"Life's one constant growth spurt when you're young like you," she said. Her eyes were all shiny as if made of glass. "I'm afraid I've grown so old the reverse is happening to me. I've started shrinking, would you believe?"

"I think you're the perfect height," I said. "Easily transportable."

She laughed then, properly loud, like it came from deep inside her belly.

"Did you know her well?" she asked me.

"Know who well?"

"Why, Ursula, of course. Ursula Grimsworth?" She gestured around the room, at the guests, the food, all of it.

"Ah." I hesitated, about to grab a handful of miniature sausage rolls. What *was* our backstory again?

Whenever Morag and I went to a funeral, we always had a backstory. The trouble was, it changed every time. It got a bit confusing remembering which story went with which funeral.

"Morag!" I remembered out loud. "Yes, Morag. Morag knew her. Morag knew her *really, really well*."

"Morag?"

"Yes, Morag's my mum. She was a … distant niece of Mrs Grimsworth," I recited, just as we'd practised on the bus on the journey there. "They were *estranged*."

Morag always told me to use the word *estranged*. It freaked people out, apparently. Made them stop asking questions.

"*Hmph*, how bizarre." The old lady raised a thin, pencilled eyebrow. "I didn't think Ursula had any family to speak of."

"Oh, yes," I said, nodding. "Morag loved her very much, and they spent *lots* of time together."

I swallowed and glanced nervously at Morag across the room, to check she wasn't spying on me like she sometimes did.

I watched as she not-so-sneakily tipped an entire plate of ham-and-cheese sandwich triangles into the empty plastic tub she kept inside her handbag. Nobody saw her, but she needed to be more careful.

I turned back to the old woman. "They used to spend Christmas together every year!" I blurted out of nowhere, trying to stop her from looking over and noticing Morag.

"Is that so? But I thought you said they were estranged?"

"Um, yes..." I swallowed. I did say they were estranged, but that didn't mean I actually had any idea what *estranged* meant.

Morag said I wasn't any good at keeping secrets,

but I knew that wasn't true, because I'd kept so many secrets for her. She always said I'd sell my deepest, darkest secret for a chicken nugget, given half a chance.

"They used to send each other cards and presents too," I said, the words pouring out of my mouth uncontrollably like sick. "Every birthday, Christmas and sometimes Easter!"

The old lady's face dropped its polite smile and shifted into a deeply wrinkled, concerned frown. I often had that effect on people. Suddenly she didn't seem so friendly any more.

"Well, I must acquaint myself with this so-called *niece Morag*," she sputtered. "I find it difficult to believe that Ursula never mentioned her to me, not once in forty-seven years of friendship and embroidery club!"

"Oh, that is strange." I felt my face starting to glow.

The lady put down her plate and scoured the crowd. Morag, perfectly timed, slipped between two groups of chatting mourners and disappeared into the milling crowd. Dressed in black, she blended in perfectly.

"Curious," the lady said. "Very curious."

I felt the blood draining from my head like somebody had pulled the plug out of me. Was she on to us? Did she know that Morag and I hadn't been invited?

"Anyway, I should go." I pointed to the bathroom.

"I'd better see where my mum has got to. She'll be worried about me."

"Indeed." She scowled. "Indeed you had."

I felt the old lady's eyes glaring into the back of my head as I shuffled away and merged into the mass of people. I needed to tell Morag that somebody was on to us.

Morag always vanished somehow. One minute she was right in front of you, the next she was gone without a trace. It happened everywhere: the supermarket, the beach, the bus station in town. She should have been a magician. I would try not to panic, but the longer she was gone, the more my head started to pound.

It was even worse when she did a disappearing act at a funeral. Trying to distinguish Morag from the countless grown-ups in drab black funeral outfits was practically impossible. Often I would hear her cackling laugh before I saw her, but now I couldn't hear that either.

I checked everywhere: outside the ladies' toilets, inside the ladies' toilets, in the wet and stinky smoking area, under the little kids' slide out in the pub garden. She wasn't even in the seating area where she'd said she would be.

Just when I was about to give up, I found her at

precisely the last place I wanted her to be: the bar. A weird feeling trickled from my head and down to my toes. This wasn't good.

I watched as Morag picked a glass of wine from a teetering pyramid of glasses that was stacked on the counter. Then, opening her throat like the pelicans I'd seen on the telly, she tipped it right to the back of her neck without even tasting it.

"Morag?" I tugged on the back of her leather jacket.

"Solo!" she said, so loudly that a few people turned and looked. She planted a big sloppy kiss on my cheek, probably leaving a lipstick stain like always. "Solo, my beautiful, darling boy. Are you having fun? This is a good one, don't you think?"

"No, Morag," I whispered. "I'm not having fun. And *be quiet*. You're talking really loud."

"Oh, shush, you," she gabbled. "Don't be so *boring* for once! You always try to act so perfect. Your mother's having some fun. You ought to try it sometime!"

"You don't understand," I said under my breath. "Somebody *knows*, Morag."

"You what? Somebody knows what?" She stumbled back and nearly knocked over a bar stool. It rocked on its long legs like a basketball circling the hoop.

"Oh, nearly lost my balance there!" she said,

laughing. "It's these silly boots. Honestly, I'll wear my trainers next time!"

"Stop it, Morag," I whispered angrily. "Somebody knows we're not supposed to be here."

Morag burst out in fake, loud laughter. "Of course we're supposed to be here, darling. I'm here commiserating the loss of my dear aunt Caroline, or whatever her blimmin' name is!"

"It's Ursula Grimsworth," I hissed. "You know it is. This old lady started chatting to me, and she knows. She *knows*, Morag."

"Well, what on earth did you say to her?" Morag leaned in close so her face was next to mine. "We've practised this routine, Solo. Plenty of times. What exactly did you say?"

"I said you were her niece," I said, my voice going high and defensive.

"Really?" Morag narrowed her eyes at me. "That's really all you said?"

"And that you sometimes spent Christmas and Easter together. That's all. I promise that's all I said to her!"

Morag sighed and covered her face with her hands. "I told you to say I was her *estranged* niece, Solo. What didn't you understand about *estranged*?"

I shrugged. I had no idea what to say. I'd ruined another funeral. There was no telling how long it would take for Morag to forgive me this time.

"Well, I suppose that's that, then," Morag said. She did up her handbag more aggressively than usual. "I suppose we'd better leave before they *make* us leave."

"I'm sorry—" I began.

"Save it," Morag hissed. "We'll just have to try again tomorrow."

Across the room I spotted the old lady from the buffet. She was watching Morag's and my every move, slowly shaking her head.

Morag took my hand, turned and dragged me quickly towards the exit. She paused, momentarily, then grabbed a glass of white wine from a tray by the door.

"One for the road," she gasped, gulping it down. "Now let's get out of here."

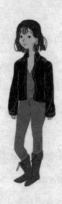

CHAPTER 2

Morag was in a really bad mood after I almost got us caught. She didn't say one word to me on the entire walk to the bus stop. Whenever I tried to speak, she ignored me.

Morag got in a mood like this sometimes. She had a special name for it: the Big Bad Reds, or the BBRs for short. Apparently, an evil red mist would descend into her eyes, and all she could see was how rubbish the whole world was.

Whenever Morag was suffering from the BBRs, her voice went snappy and the words she used didn't sound anything like the real her. Words that would get me a demerit at school if I got caught using them. If she wasn't using bad words, she was totally silent.

We'd learned about mental health a bit at school, but it was still confusing. There were so many words like *depression* and *anxiety* floating around, but I wasn't sure whether that's what Morag had. All I knew was that some of her moods were trickier than others.

Her face changed too. Her eyes bulged, her skin went red. The vein in her forehead stuck out like it was about to explode. When I was little I thought she would turn into an actual dragon. Now that I'm older, I know that wasn't true.

"*Another dreaded case of the Big Bad Reds,*" she would say, once she'd calmed down and was trying to make everything better again. Then she would start going on at me not to tell anyone in case I got taken away to live in a home.

I'd got used to the BBRs over the ten years of my life. Whether they lasted a few hours or a few days, I knew she'd always go back to normal eventually. I supposed Morag couldn't help it, even if there were moments when I thought she could try a bit harder.

In the meantime, I tried to remind myself about that thing people say about sticks and stones not breaking bones, and names not hurting either. Morag would never throw a stick or a stone – that's all that mattered.

After the Reds were over, she would start apologizing, telling me how she hadn't really meant it, saying sorry and *"You know I love you very much, don't you?"* over and over again until I would get annoyed and catch the Big Bad Reds myself. The Reds were contagious, just like a stuffy nose.

That's exactly what happened at the bus stop after we almost got caught. Morag kept staring at me, then looking away all upset. Then she would look back at me, just to see whether I was looking at her.

We'd missed the bus when we got there, so I had to put up with a good twenty-five minutes of Morag chain-smoking rollies and apologizing and calling herself a terrible witch on a never-ending loop.

"That was a close one, Solo," she said, exhaling cigarette smoke, which the breeze whipped away. Her hand, covered in her special gold rings, was shaking. "We should come up with a better backstory next time."

"It's fine, Morag," I sighed. "It was all my fault."

I felt like the red embarrassed face on the "Emotions and Feelings" poster at school. I couldn't look Morag in the eye, so I stared into the distance, pretending I was someone else.

This was one of my favourite hobbies. I would

imagine myself in a nice posh house. There was a driveway at the front and a conker tree in the garden. There'd be a cat and a dog and a mum with blonde shiny hair and an apron complete with flour stains from all the delicious cakes she was constantly baking for me. There was a dad who could teach me football and take me to get my hair cut at an actual barber's shop instead of doing my fringe in the kitchen. Then there was my little brother, or sister, who was practically obsessed with me, always wanting to play games and hang out. I even had a mountain bike, and a huge gaming set-up with multiple screens and—

Morag elbowed me in the side, as if we were suddenly best mates again. She did this whenever she was trying to cheer me up.

"You know you're my favourite son in the whole wide world, right?" She started trying to tickle me under my arms. Even though I didn't find it funny, I started laughing.

"I'm your *only* son," I replied with a smirk. "I'm your only child, full stop."

"That's why I called you Solo." She winked. "Because you're the only one I'll ever need. You, my fine young man, are the cream of the crop!"

I nodded, even though she said that all the time.

She loved telling me again and again why exactly she gave me such an embarrassing name. Sometimes I told people it's short for Solomon, but it isn't. It even says it on my birth certificate – *Given name(s): Solo.*

"There he is, my happy boy!" She laughed. "All's well that ends well when it comes to family. And that's what we are, Solo: a *family.*"

"All's *not* well," I muttered, remembering I was supposed to be annoyed. "I don't want to go to funerals any more." A motorbike roared past so Morag didn't hear the last bit.

"Here, have a look at this," she whispered, opening her handbag.

Inside was the plastic tub she carried everywhere, stuffed with all the best bits of the funeral food that she'd swiped. Ham-and-cheese sandwiches, sausage rolls, cheese and pineapple chunks on pointy wooden sticks.

"Not bad, eh? All wasn't lost. Feast Night tonight!"

I smiled, but I felt a bit funny inside. I did enjoy our Feast Nights… I just wished we didn't have to go to funerals to get the food for the feast. Why couldn't we just go to the supermarket and fill up a trolley like everyone else?

I already knew why: money. There was never

enough of it. Even the child benefit Morag got every month didn't help much. Money was stretched so thin it was almost see through.

On Feast Nights, we'd sit on cushions on the floor and spread out the funeral food like a picnic. Sometimes, Morag would add extra treats like chicken nuggets and hash browns, and we'd eat until our stomachs stuck out like pigs. Recently, I'd started to feel weird about it though. I knew that not everyone had Feast Nights like Morag and me, and Morag told me to keep it secret.

"Did you manage to get much?" she asked. "Any spoils to add to the feast?"

I shook my head. "Didn't get a chance. That old lady started talking to me and she knew what we were doing." I felt the embarrassment over again. "I lost my plate when I came to find you."

Morag's face fell. "Oh, right. That isn't ideal. Maybe Derek at the corner shop will loan me another pizza on the sly. What do you fancy? Pepperoni?"

I hated it when Morag did that. She would drag me to the shop and ask to have food and drink without paying for it. She would wheel me out like the DVD player at school, pretend that I was starving or something, and beg the shopkeeper for whatever she could get. She always promised to pay them back. Customers would line up behind us, tutting, wondering what was taking so long.

"The bus is here, Morag," I said, pointing down the road.

A red double-decker was rounding the corner towards us. I spent half my life on buses, being dragged from one funeral to the next, all over south London, but I was grateful to change the subject.

Morag perked up. "Brilliant, we'll be home in no time!" She leaned towards me, as if to share an exciting secret. "Now listen, I've not got the fare. Play along."

"Morag, no!" I protested.

The double doors of the bus parted with a mechanical hiss, and Morag strode up to where the driver was seated.

"I'm *so* sorry to do this," she said, putting on her most respectable posh voice. "I'm mortified, honestly. I've been mugged, you see. These two hooded youths approached on bikes and snatched my purse and all my money clean out of my hands! So me and my son here –" she gestured towards me – "can't get home."

"You sound like you've been through the wars today," said the driver. "It's no bother to me, love. On you get."

"Oh, thank you. Thank you so much." Morag practically curtseyed. "You *are* a kind soul. People like you restore my faith in humanity!"

Morag made her way to the upper deck, her heels clattering on the stairs.

The driver nodded at me with pity as I skulked aboard behind Morag. I kept my mouth shut, not wanting to add to the mountain of lies that was already piling up in the back of my mind.

We sat on the very front seat on the top deck, which was my favourite. I always sat there so I could see into other people's houses and imagine what their lives were like. The windows were steamy, so I smeared a lookout hole in the condensation.

A few minutes into the journey Morag started, as if she'd snapped out of a distant dream. She rummaged for a second, and then produced a small, scrunched-up sandwich bag from her jacket pocket.

"What am I like? I almost forgot this!" She put the warm, clear bag in my hands and I realized it was a load of breaded mozzarella dippers that she'd swiped from the funeral.

They were a little bit squished, and some of the cheesy filling was leaking out from being stuffed in Morag's pocket. But I still wanted them. How could I not?

I pierced a hole in the bag with my thumb and shoved one of the sticks into my mouth, savouring the cheesy taste oozing between my teeth as I chomped.

"They're still warm," I said through a mouthful. "Thanks, Morag."

She smiled back at me. "Plenty more where that came from, kid."

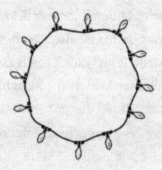

CHAPTER 3

We were soaked with rain by the time we got back to the flat. Morag's wonky fringe (which she chopped herself with the kitchen scissors, usually after she'd done mine) clung to her forehead in thick strands. The raindrops danced on the surface of her leather jacket.

My black funeral suit was sopping. The soaked fabric clung tight to my legs like cold wet tissue. Morag said it didn't matter though, because it would dry overnight on the radiator.

I hated that scratchy old suit. Morag got it from the men's rail of a charity shop ages ago. It was so big that the sleeves had to be rolled up twice, and the trouser legs hung down over my shoes, making me look as if I had hooves. Even though I'd worn the suit to loads of funerals, it felt as though it never belonged to me. It was like bringing someone else's jumper home from school by accident. It just didn't feel right.

Morag made me take off the saggy suit and put on my pyjamas, while she got into her polka-dot dressing gown. Next, she hung my suit over the radiators in the main hallway. Morag didn't want to waste money, so she always hung our clothes to dry in the communal area where the heating was free. Even pants and socks with grubby stains were hung out for all the neighbours to stare at.

I knew posh Mr Thurston from across the hall must have hated seeing our underwear drying out there. I'd seen him tutting at our clothes and shaking his head when I watched him through the spyhole. He *owned* his flat, so he was more fussy about things. Ours was rented, but recently Morag had started telling me not to open the door to the landlord.

We could tell that Mr Thurston was posh from a mile off. He was always coming and going in a smart blue suit and carrying a leather briefcase. He had sporty-looking car in the shared car park, with an alarm so sensitive it screamed if you just looked at it.

He was always getting packages delivered from the internet. Every day something new would arrive.

Some in huge boxes, some in tiny ones. Whenever he wasn't home, Morag had to take his packages instead. Sometimes our front door was buried in his cardboard boxes. Morag got sick of it after a while and stopped answering the door, full stop.

Morag always told me not to speak to Mr Thurston. Morag didn't like me talking to any grown-ups really, in case I got us into trouble with my mouth.

The flat was dark and horrible that night, as though no one lived there. Cold air was creeping in through the windows, along with the blue lights of police cars and the whine and noise of rushing traffic.

"Right, how about I spruce things up in here, then?" Morag said, reading my mind. "Nice bit of ambiance for Feast Night."

She pulled the curtains shut and switched on all the twinkling strings of fairy lights. She also lit the tealight candles she kept dotted around. In no time, the living room felt like a cosy grotto full of warm light, where nothing bad could happen at all.

Next, Morag took all the cushions off the sofa and the pillows off our beds and placed them in a circle in the middle of the living-room floor. Then she brought in her double duvet and wrapped it round my shoulders for extra cosiness. The last few raindrops escaped from my hair and snaked down my neck. My toes started to feel nice and warm. They tingled like pins and needles as they came back to life.

She brought in plates and spread them out in the middle of the floor. Finally, she unboxed all the funeral food, laying it out neatly.

It was an OK selection, but nothing compared to some of the stuff we'd got before. Sometimes they had hot food at funerals as well as cold nibbles. Stuff like lasagnes, pasta bakes, chips. If you lingered for an hour or two until the other guests had gone, it was easier to spoon bigger portions into plastic lunchboxes and squirrel it away. I know some people say it's bad to steal food, but it all went in the bin otherwise.

That's what Morag said, at least. *Waste not, want not*, she always goes.

"Voilà!" Morag exclaimed, spreading her arms out as if she'd conjured up a magic trick. "Let them eat … mini ham-and-cheese sandwiches! Dig in, Solo. Fill your boots."

I tucked in right away, shoving the food into my mouth. The ham was a bit slimy, and the cheese was dry at the corners, but I still enjoyed it. I chewed and chewed, and after a while I started to feel quite full.

Morag seemed to be biting her nails more than the food.

"Why aren't you eating, Morag? Are you not hungry?"

She looked awkward and shrugged one shoulder. "Not really, darling. But you go on – eat up. As much as you can."

"But why? I thought Feast Night was for you *and* me?"

She smiled, but shook her head at the same time. "It's not a very big haul today, Solo. You're a growing lad. You need it more than I do. Eat it all up – go on."

I put another mini sausage roll into my mouth, but it didn't taste the same knowing that Morag wasn't eating too. It felt like a wodge of cardboard slowly squeezing down my throat.

"Have some, Morag," I said. I slid a couple of sandwiches on to an empty plate, and pushed it towards her. "If you don't eat too, then how will you have energy to look after me?"

She laughed, but only through her nose, not properly.

"A lot of people might say I don't look after you right as it is, Sol. They think I'm a bad mum."

"No they don't! Nobody thinks you're a bad mum.

You're ace! You're fun, you're not boring – you're different every day!"

She did the sad nose-laugh again. I knew she was in a weird mood when she did that, as though she couldn't even muster up the effort to laugh out of her mouth.

"You sound like your dad. He used to say the exact same thing. Used to call me unpredictable. A *wild card*, he called me."

I swallowed my cheese and pineapple chunks slowly. I felt uncomfortable when Morag talked about Dad. It was like reading a story with no goodies and no funny bits. Only the baddies wrecking things again and again.

I looked at Morag. "I didn't know he used to say that."

"Yeah, he sure did." She shrugged. "Used to say a lot of things like that. Wasn't enough though, oh no. I wasn't *unpredictable* enough to stop him running off with that *Imelda* woman, was I? He soon got bored of little old me, *wild card* or not."

"Morag," I said, still chewing. "Don't."

"And now they're getting married, of course. Church bells a-ringing." She rolled her eyes.

"What?" A chunk of sausage roll fell from my

mouth, leaving a trail of pastry flakes down my pyjamas.

Morag sighed. "I didn't want to tell you, Solo. I guess that's why I've been in such a rubbish mood lately."

My head started pounding. My mouth was open, but no words came out. For some reason I felt the need to smush a sandwich with my fist. I knew it was stupid, but I couldn't help it.

Morag fished around in her handbag and produced her cracked mobile phone in its scuffed leopard-print case. She was always dropping it, see. She scrolled a few times, her eyes squinting at the screen. She tossed the phone towards me as though she was throwing away a piece of rubbish.

"Here you go – look. Get a load of that."

I felt my face turn into a snarl at the sight of him. The sight of *them*.

It was a photo of my dad, his face peeking out between the cracks in the glass. He looked different. He had a golden-brown tan, and his hair was cut smart. It wasn't long and straggly like the last time I'd seen him five years ago. Beside him was Imelda, also tanned. Her horrible wide smile was painted red with stupid clown lipstick.

Imelda's hand rested on my dad's shoulder, showing off a gold ring with a glimmering clear stone. They were on a beach, somewhere sunny that didn't look like England. The sun was setting behind them, all oranges and pinks smearing into the sky.

"They're on holiday?" I said. "Abroad?"

"Oh, yes," Morag said. "Jason's quite the jet-setter now."

Dad only ever took us on holiday to Normley-on-Sea when he lived with us. We always stayed at Sunset Dunes, a caravan park near the beach. It was nice, and we always had loads of fun. But it wasn't *abroad* nice. Morag and I have been back a few times since, so it was our special place.

"Read what it says underneath." Morag rolled her eyes again.

Over the moon to call this fine lady my fiancée! #SheSaidYes

"Morag," I said, "what's a fiancée?"

"It means Imelda's about to become your *lovely new stepmummy*." Her voice had a mean sing-song sound to it. "Her and your dad will be a picture-perfect family now. Not that *we'll* get a look-in."

Morag got up and stood by the window with her arms crossed, staring out at nothing in particular.

I wanted to be sick all over the funeral feast. I wanted to run away and bury myself in my corner and wake up in a different version of today. A version where Morag was normal and Dad wasn't getting married to Evil Imelda.

Morag came back and snatched the phone from my hand. "You'll have a wedding invite coming in the post soon. Lucky you. I'll have to get you a new suit and everything. Yet more money flushed down the drain."

"I'm not going!" I threw my plate down on to a cushion. "I hate him!"

"Flashy holidays, new fiancée, glitzy engagement ring." Morag shook her head. "He's changed since way back when. He thought all that material stuff was a load of old nonsense back then. Not quite so rock and roll now, is he?"

Dad used to be alternative, apparently. That's how he and Morag first got chatting at the call centre where they both worked, because she liked his style. He was in a band and used to live on a houseboat on the canal, which Morag thought was seriously cool. They soon got married, and I was a *pleasant surprise*, as Morag put it, born after they'd only known each other for a year. Goodbye houseboat, and goodbye rock band, I suppose. Hello nappies and baby food.

By the time I was five, they'd had over six and a half years to figure out they didn't even like each other that much. Dad moved out one day with all his stuff in bin bags and boxes. That was when the Big Bad Reds got worse. Dad said we would still see each other, but obviously that never happened.

Come to think of it, it was all one big chain reaction. If Dad hadn't moved out, Morag's mental health wouldn't have got worse, then she would never have lost her job in the end, and I wouldn't have had to spend the last six months sneaking food from funerals in an old man's suit.

Anger started swelling up inside my stomach. I felt my face start to redden and my fists begin to shake. I hated thinking about that stuff.

Morag did the fake nose-laugh again. It was as though she could read my mind. "You and me both, Solo. You and me both. Anyway..." Morag clapped her hands. "Come on, then – time for bed. You've got school tomorrow, and you need to be well rested."

"I won't be able to sleep now," I protested.

"Well, try your best," she said, clearing up the plates. "If there's one piece of advice I've got for you, Solo, it's this…" Morag leaned towards me. I could faintly smell wine on her breath from the funeral. "Never trust anyone. Especially if you think you like them. *Especially* if they say they like you. You never know how people might let you down, even the good ones."

I nodded and wrapped myself up tighter in her duvet. Usually everything was fun when we put the cushions on the floor, but Morag's Big Bad Reds were rearing up for a second wind, like a defeated dragon crawling back out of a cave to fight another round.

"Morag?" I said, desperate to talk about anything other than Dad and Imelda. "We're doing coding at school tomorrow. Making websites and stuff."

Morag was so taken aback that her eyebrows almost crawled right up into her hair. "Ooh, someone's feeling *academic* all of a sudden! Well I never. You really are a little brainbox, eh?"

I shrugged. I wasn't a brainbox. If I had to be some sort of box, I was an empty box. I wasn't really looking forward to school, but I had a feeling that Morag's bad mood would be here to stay for a while. School was the only place I could think of to escape them for a bit.

"Maybe you can make a website to track down Dad and Imelda," she joked. "Get me some of that child-support money he promised."

Now I was the one doing the fake nose-laugh. "I'd better get to bed."

"Are you sure you've had enough to eat? I think there's some tempura prawns knocking about in my handbag…"

"I'm sure," I said, standing up. The thought of handbag prawns made me feel queasy.

"You're sure you're sure?"

"Surely sure I'm sure," I said with a nod. It was a little thing we did, just us two.

"Well, come on, get comfy. You'll have an early start in the morning."

I took myself to the corner of the living room, where my mattress was tucked into my alcove between the sofa and the wall. It wasn't a real bedroom, because we only had one, and that belonged to Morag. But the sofa created a corner so it felt quite separate. I really liked my alcove, but Morag told me not to talk about it in front of other people. She said it made people feel weird.

Morag let me stick whatever I wanted on my wall. It was plastered with pictures, leaflets and drawings that I'd collected since I was little. My favourite was the photograph of Morag and me at Sunset Dunes in Normley-on-Sea, the first time we went without Dad. Morag was in a mood most of the time, but she'd started to cheer up by the end. In the photo, we're sticking our heads through specially placed holes in a painted underwater scene. I looked like an old-fashioned diver in a metal suit. Morag looked like an octopus with tentacles all covered in suckers. That was two summers ago now. I doubted we'd be going back again until Morag found another job, and that wasn't exactly going well.

After I'd slipped beneath my duvet, Morag stuck her head over the top of the sofa so she was peering down on me, like when I was a baby in a cot.

"Goodnight, Morag." I plumped my pillow into a mound. My eyes started to feel heavy, as if they were begging me to let them close.

"You're my favourite son, you know," she said softly. "The only one I'll ever need. That's why I called you—"

"Solo." I smiled.

Morag ruffled my hair and turned away. I closed my eyes and listened to the people chatting on the TV. Famous actors talking about a new film or something. I got warmer and heavier until I could almost feel dreams knocking at the door of my mind.

That's when I heard the jangle of keys and the front door slamming shut. High-heeled footsteps clattered loudly down the stairs.

"Morag?" I called into the half-dark. "Are you still there?"

There was no reply.

I pulled my duvet up to my neck. Morag was only going to the shop to get drinks for another of her parties for one; she'd be back in a minute. Sometimes Morag found enough money for certain things, even though she said she didn't have any.

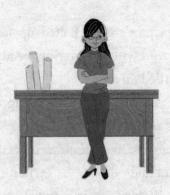

CHAPTER 4

"Melissa Underwood?"

"Yes, Miss Carmichael."

"Good morning, Melissa. Jack Vaughan?"

"Yes, Miss Carmichael."

"Good morning, Jack. Solo Walker?"

Sometimes my voice just wouldn't come out, even if I tried to force it.

Miss Carmichael's pen scratched loudly as she drew a red cross next to my name on the register. Everybody in the whole classroom started to giggle.

"Yes, Miss," I finally murmured. I raised my hand quickly before it shot straight back down into my pocket like a meerkat retreating into a hole. My face went red and hot like the rings on top of the oven.

Miss Carmichael's head bolted up fast, and she scanned the room with her glaring, beady eyes until finally they settled on me.

"Ah, there you are," she said, rising to her feet. "Taken a bit of artistic licence with the uniform again, have we?" She smiled, but I couldn't tell if it was a kind smile or a mean one.

Everybody giggled again, and I went redder. Everybody's eyes pressed on my skin like fingers. I pulled my jumper sleeves down over my hands, but they were too short because I'd been wearing it for years. My wrists stuck out like the bones on two roast chicken drumsticks.

"Those trousers, that jumper, that suit jacket. I'm afraid that's going to be another demerit. I'll let you off for this week to get it sorted, but any longer than that and I will have to send a letter home."

Miss Carmichael was confusing. She had a knack for being horrible and nice at the same time. If she liked you, it was easy to tell. You would be selected to write on the whiteboard in lessons and got extra privileges at break time. If she really liked you, you would be awarded the Star of the Week, which meant you got to wear a shiny gold star pin badge and go first in the lunch line.

I had never been Star of the Week because Miss Carmichael didn't like me at all. I didn't like her either, so I suppose we were even.

Miss Carmichael crossed the classroom, her shoes squeaking on the floor, and placed a round red sticker on the laminated chart behind me. I blinked hard. The trail of red stickers next to my name stretched miles longer than anybody else's. It even snaked round the edges of the chart where I was starting to run out of room.

I did have a couple of green stickers too, for times when I'd been good. One for when I found a caterpillar in the playground, picked it up and put it in a tree to keep it from getting squished by the boys playing football. Another for handing in Melissa Underwood's missing capybara plushie that I found by the bins, covered in mud and dust.

Nobody knew it was actually me who'd put the capybara in the bin in the first place, because Melissa Underwood was the worst person in the whole class. I certainly wasn't going to tell Miss Carmichael.

"Let's try to get this uniform sorted, shall we?" Miss Carmichael said to me quietly. "How about I give you some information after class for you to pass on to your mum? Everything she needs to know about uniforms, and how we can help. Does that sound OK?"

I kept my mouth zipped tight like Morag's leather jacket. Miss Carmichael absolutely loved trick questions. Most of the time it didn't matter if you answered *yes*, *no* or *thirty-seven* – she wasn't ever happy. Well, at least not where I was concerned.

"That's a lesson to you all," she said, squeaking back to her seat at the front. "I know it's boring, but wearing the correct school uniform teaches us an invaluable life lesson about rules and order, even if it does feel like a bit of a pain sometimes."

"I wouldn't want to dress like *him*, anyway," hissed Kai Bailey from across the class. "He's proper *weird*."

The gang of boys sitting at Kai's table struggled to hide their smirks. Miss Carmichael didn't seem to hear. I shot my most vicious scowl their way, but it only made them laugh more.

Miss Carmichael finished the register, then turned to the board and started writing stuff about coding in red marker. My eyes went blurry and I gave up trying to concentrate almost as soon as Miss Carmichael had started.

Instead I daydreamed about what I would do if I had powers. I imagined I could turn Miss Carmichael and Kai Bailey into giant chickens right there in front of everyone in the classroom. They would gobble and cluck, and peck at seeds in a mucky trough. They'd scratch their scrawny chicken feet into the ground—

"Any thoughts, Solo?" Miss Carmichael asked, shattering my daydream into a million little shards. "What do we know about Python?"

"Uhm." I gulped. "They strangle their prey and swallow it up whole, don't they?"

Everybody laughed again.

Miss Carmichael rolled her eyes. "Very funny, ha ha. Do try to stay with us, Solo."

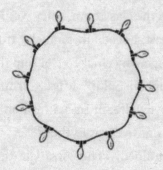

CHAPTER 5

"Ooh, here he is," Morag said when she heard the door slam shut behind me. "My little coding wizard! They were saying there's a *lot* of money in coding on the telly earlier."

She was cleaning the kitchen, making it look like Feast Night and the party for one never happened. She always cleaned after the Big Bad Reds, as if cleaning up in the real world somehow cleaned up the mess inside her head too. My heart sank as I noticed she was wearing her funeral clothes again.

"I hate coding. I hate all of it."

I dumped my bag in the corner of the hallway and dropped my jacket on the floor. I'd already decided I didn't want to talk about it. How could I explain that I'd got a demerit, been laughed at *and* humiliated in front of everyone, just in one day?

"Look at you, all sweetness and light," Morag said sarcastically. "It can't be that bad, can it?"

"I don't want to talk about it," I grumbled, as rehearsed.

"Oh, go on." Morag appeared beside me. "It might help. I thought you were looking forward to coding."

"It isn't as fun as I thought it would be."

"Well, school isn't worth the trouble, if you ask me," Morag said. "They grind you down, get rid of all your individuality and that. They make out that education is the only important thing in life, but look at me. I hardly ever went to school and I turned out fine!"

The kitchen bin was overflowing with empty bottles and cans and rubbish. The leftover food from the stolen feast was in the fridge to keep it fresh. I grabbed a handful of mini sandwiches and melted into the sofa. I patted around for the remote and turned on the telly.

The sandwiches didn't taste good any more. The bread was dry and the ham was even slimier than before. Still, I chewed and chewed, imagining with each mouthful I was chomping on the heads of Miss Cowmichael, Melissa, Ameyo, Mina, Kai Bailey and his gang that followed him around.

"Are you sure that's what's the matter?" Morag said without looking up from her cleaning. "You've come in like a right old storm cloud."

"I got a demerit again," I said, flicking through the channels.

"Not again! What for? I swear that Miss Carmichael must have it in for you…" Morag trailed off.

"For my uniform. My trousers aren't right, the jacket isn't right. I've had this ratty old jumper since I was about seven!"

Morag stopped wiping the worktop and rolled her eyes. "You weren't *seven*. Don't be so dramatic. You must've been about eight, something like that."

There wasn't anything good on the telly. Just posh grown-ups sitting around desks talking about boring things happening in the world. I switched it off and stared into the dusty black screen.

Morag was watching me. "Is that really the reason Miss Carmichael keeps giving you all these demerits?" She stood with one hand on her hip, the other holding a dripping yellow cloth.

"*Yes!*" I said, louder than I'd meant to. "I've told you before: it has to be exactly the right uniform or it doesn't count."

"But you look nice and smart in your suit!"

"None of the other kids *wear* suits, Morag! They wear normal school uniform with the proper logo on, from the uniform shop like everyone else!"

"Well, why would you want to be like everyone else? Life would be so boring if everyone looked the same all the time, wouldn't it?"

I closed my eyes because I was getting angry, and getting angry made everything even worse. I said things I regretted when I was angry, then I'd have to go crawling back to Morag for forgiveness.

"Can I please just have a proper uniform, Morag?" My teeth were clenched. "Miss Carmichael's going to send a letter home if I get two more demerits."

Morag smirked. "Who does she think she is, the Royal Mail? She can send all the letters she likes, but she's not my teacher. She can't tell me what to do. If she thinks she can, she's got another think coming."

"She says there's grants!"

"*Pfft*, grants." Morag shook her head. "I don't *need* grants. I'm going to get everything sorted."

I got up from the sofa and slumped down on to my mattress. I wouldn't win this argument with Morag. I never won *any* arguments with Morag. She hated being told what to do, and she hated Miss Cowmichael even more than I did.

In fact, I'm pretty sure it was Morag who came up with that nickname after I got detention for sneaking on to the coach trip to Cadbury World. Morag said forty-five quid was too much money just for me to go and look at some chocolate she could buy in the corner shop down the street. I was supposed to spend the day helping the school receptionist, but when the coach turned up I couldn't help myself but get on board before everyone else. I knew someone would find me and kick me off, but I just wanted to feel like I was going too for a few seconds. Soon everybody else got on board and the engine started to rumble. I knew I should stand up and tell someone I was there, but I didn't. When we started to drive out of the car park I got this massive adrenaline rush.

I only stayed hidden for about fifteen minutes in the end. I would've got away with it if Ameyo hadn't shrieked when she found me hiding beneath two empty seats at the back. No Cadbury World for me.

Morag poked her head over the back of the sofa and looked at me. I rolled over and faced the wall. She didn't get the hint.

"Look, I'll try, OK?" she sighed. "I'll try to get you the proper uniform with the logos and all that nonsense. And guess what – I've had some pretty good news that might just help with that."

Morag had a mischievous glint in her eye and was struggling to keep a straight face.

"What?" I rolled back to face her properly. "What news?"

"I've only gone and got an interview!" She leaped off the sofa and did a little dance on the spot, pumping her fists into the air. "Friday morning at ten o'clock."

"Seriously? That's amazing! What's it for?"

"*Bojangles*," she said, in her posh-lady voice. "That nice clothes shop on the main road. *Bojangles offers a curated selection of up-and-coming designer garments for cosmopolitan women.* That's what the website says, anyway. I'd only be folding clothes, sprucing up the displays. *Your receipt's in the bag*, that type of stuff. I've got a good feeling about this one!"

"You're going to do amazing, Morag," I said, sitting up. "When did you find out?"

"Today, when you were at school. They called me up. They sounded so friendly and nice. Just between us, I reckon it might just be a formality, this interview."

"That's amazing! I know you're going to smash this one, Morag. You've always wanted to work at Bojangles."

"Well, I'll give it my best damn shot. I can just imagine it: me, folding all the … *garments*, I suppose they'd call them. Making the window display look nice at Christmas. It'll be loads more glam than that grotty old ticket office at the train station, that's for sure."

Morag used to work at the train station, printing out people's tickets and telling them which train went where. She liked it at first, but it didn't work out. Every interview she'd had since hadn't worked out. Morag said that if she received one more email saying *unfortunately you were unsuccessful on this occasion*, she was liable to explode.

She'd had jobs before, but none of them had ever lasted. She'd worked in shops, in a factory, then at the train station. Sometimes Morag kept hold of the job for a while and even said she enjoyed it. But things always went wrong somehow. Either the job got sick of Morag, or Morag got sick of the job.

Now that I was thinking about it, I realized that's when everything started to go wrong for Morag and me. When she lost that final job a few months back, everything changed, and Morag was never the same. The money troubles only made her worse.

Then my shoes started getting small, and my uniform started getting ropey. Food started costing too much, and it got harder to make a meal out of the money she had. Then it cost too much to keep the flat nice and warm. That's when we started going to funerals with our pockets lined with food bags and Morag's handbag prepped with empty boxes.

"Good luck, Morag." I slumped back on to my pillow. "If it doesn't work out, you can always ask Dad for the money." I knew it was a silly thing to say, but it came out anyway.

Morag smirked. "Thanks for the vote of confidence, Solo. Of course it'll work out. I think I'm overdue a bit of good luck, don't you?"

I nodded. We were both overdue a bit of luck.

"Right then, come on. Seeing as you're home nice and early, let's get a wiggle on and zip to this funeral."

"Oh, Morag, do we have to?" I moaned. "I'm really not in the mood."

"Yes," Morag said, already pacing the flat, searching

for her bag and black coat. "Mood or not, the fridge is still pretty empty, unless you haven't noticed? Plus, it'll be nice to get out of the flat for a bit."

"Fine," I grumbled.

"Cheer up, Solo." Morag was smiling. "If my interview goes to plan, this could well be one of the last funerals we ever have to go to!"

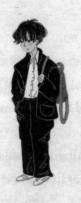

CHAPTER 6

The crematorium was set behind two huge black metal gates, like some sort of posh mansion or something. We'd never been to this crematorium before, so Morag was excited. It was miles out from home, almost in the countryside. It didn't feel like London at all. Morag loved the look of it. She kept grabbing my hand and going, "Isn't it nice, Solo? Isn't it *classy*?"

As we trudged down the gravelled crematorium driveway, black funeral cars passed by slowly in an endless parade. This was loads fancier than the funerals we normally snuck into. My stomach rippled with nervousness.

Everything looked proper smart and elegant. The building was practically a castle, and the gardens were like something I'd only seen in films about kings and queens in the olden days. Soft, bouncy grass. Neat hedges trimmed into animal shapes. Real-life peacocks roaming around, showing off their shimmering tail feathers.

Morag and I looked out of place compared to everyone else, making our way down the gravel drive on foot while they arrived in style. People stared at us as they rolled past, probably wondering who we were and why we weren't riding in a Rolls-Royce like them.

"Morag…" I squeezed her gloved hand tight. "Everyone's looking at us funny."

"And?" She cocked an eyebrow. "It's a free country – they can gawp at us as much as they like. For all they know, our chauffeur-driven limousine broke down en route." She waved at a passing car, but nobody waved back. "We could even be *millionaires*!"

"What's *on root*?" We weren't posh enough to be here, let alone to be speaking French. "They're *really* staring – look!"

"Well, maybe they like your suit. Or my outfit!"

I looked down at the sagging black suit with damp rain patches. The trouser legs were soaking up the puddles from the driveway. They were *not* admiring my suit.

"I don't like this, Morag. I feel weird."

"Listen to me. It's all about acting natural." Morag stopped and held my wrists. "Hold your head up high, like you *deserve* to be here. Follow me." She walked ahead, holding her head high like a giraffe, peering down her nose in the way that posh people do. "It's *easy*!"

I copied Morag's walk, holding my head as high as I could stretch it. I almost started to forget we were just pretending. I started to feel as though we belonged here. As though we belonged anywhere we wanted.

The people began exiting their cars and gathering outside the chapel. They looked sorrowful. I felt bad for them, seeing them all upset. I'd never known anyone that had actually died, but coming to all these funerals with Morag had taught me it was one of the saddest, hardest things in the world.

Morag and I had probably been to thirty funerals by then, and every one of them was as sad as the one before. Even those where people wore bright colours and had a big party, with dancing. There was always a sadness that somebody special wouldn't be around any more.

The saddest funerals felt a bit like watching the last-ever episode of your favourite TV show. There was this stinging, horrible feeling that grew bigger and bigger in your throat, knowing that there would never be any more episodes again. At the same time there was this warm feeling when you realized you could always rewatch the old episodes and relive the memories.

The two of us lingered at the back of the queue while we waited to go in. Morag told me not to stand too close and to look at the ground, in case someone asked us a question and I let the cat out the bag again.

Suddenly the crowd gasped and turned at once, and we saw a massive black carriage being pulled down the driveway by four huge black horses. I had never seen a carriage so big; it was like something from a film.

"Wow," I said without thinking. "That's so cool!"

Morag elbowed me to shush.

Inside was a wooden coffin with gold metal handles running down the edges. Surrounding it were the brightest, most tropical-looking flowers I'd ever seen in my whole life. Oranges, blues, pinks. Some of the flowers spelled out words like DAD and HUSBAND and BEST FRIEND. Others were gathered in the shape of a football. At the back of the carriage, an arrangement said: STRIKER.

Most of the people started crying at the sight of it. The women put their heads on the men's shoulders, leaving creamy make-up marks on their suit jackets. The men pulled crumpled tissues out of the ends of their sleeves and tried to keep their feelings locked in.

I suddenly felt bad for being there. This was a private thing, and I wanted to go home. I didn't tell Morag that, though, because she would only have told me off. After all, we needed the funeral food.

Morag didn't look upset. She gawped as the horses and carriage went past us, the horses' hooves sending gravel clattering around our feet. I could read Morag's mind. She thought it looked expensive and impressive. She was trying to figure out how much the carriage and shiny black coffin had cost. Guessing the price was Morag's favourite game.

The chapel doors opened, and we followed the crowd inside to the sound of classical music.

"Come on, Solo – let's make sure we get a good seat," Morag whispered. "And remember: don't talk to *anyone*. We don't need them sniffing us out."

After we sat down, six smartly dressed men entered the chapel. They were shuddering under the weight of the coffin that was resting on their shoulders. I stared at the ground, wishing I was somewhere else.

As the doors closed behind us, locking everyone in, Morag took a quick swig from a small metal flask she conjured from her handbag. "That should liven things up a bit," she said.

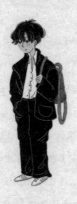

CHAPTER 7

The funeral service was just like usual. Lots of "dearly departed" and "dust to dust", whatever that meant. During the readings I picked at a loose thread on my jacket sleeve, trying to free the button on the right cuff. Maybe if the button fell off, Morag would get me my uniform.

Meanwhile, everyone else sang hymns and kept standing up and sitting down at the command of the vicar. Sad music played on and off, and lots of people were crying.

It dawned on me halfway through that the man whose funeral this was must have been a pretty big deal. I turned over the booklet I'd been given – the "Order of Service", it was called. On the front was a photo of a man in a football kit, holding a big shiny metal trophy. Underneath, the caption read:

CELEBRATING THE LIFE OF MARTIN WINNER
AKA "THE LUCKY STRIKER"
(1945–2024)

He must have been a famous footballer in the olden days, like one from the World Cup or something. He looked proper strong and muscly in the photo, with a gleaming set of straight white teeth like only famous people have.

There were more photos inside the booklet too, including one of him wearing a funny knitted jumper and flared trousers with high platform shoes. In another photo he had a blond spiky haircut and wore a jacket with shoulder pads. He must have been into fancy dress or something, because he'd had so many different outfits over the years.

The final photo was of the same man, with the same straight white glinting teeth, only loads older. His face was granddad-like and crumpled, like a receipt from the bottom of Morag's handbag. He was in a hospital bed with tubes going in and out of his nose, but he was still smiling and doing a thumbs up, even though he probably felt as rough as stale bread.

After a few more hymns, some red curtains closed round the coffin, and the funeral was over. The vicar said guests were welcome to join the family at a catered event at the Queen's Head pub nearby. Morag squeezed my leg. I shuffled away, embarrassed.

Everyone slowly left the chapel to the sound of sad music. Outside they stood around shaking hands and saying things like, "Lovely service," and, "Exactly what he would've wanted." I nodded along, but I didn't know Martin Winner at all, let alone what he *would've wanted*.

The hanging around afterwards was my least favourite part of a funeral, because you never knew how long it would take. Sometimes it took an hour for everyone to shake hands and make their way to the buffet. We had to wait for them to be done, otherwise it would look weird if Morag and I arrived first. We needed to blend into the crowd, not stand out.

"That was a good one, eh?" Morag said, slipping the order of service into her handbag. She would add it to her collection later, no doubt. "He must have been a celebrity or something. I have a feeling we'll be eating well today, Solo. This should be quite the catered wake."

My stomach started rumbling then, right on time. I started thinking about chicken nuggets and garlic bread and sausage rolls and all the funeral food that was waiting for us. My mouth even started watering a bit.

Rain started to pepper us in fat dollops, and the rest of the funeral-goers opened their black umbrellas and scattered into their fancy cars. We stood there while the flecks of rain danced off Morag's leather jacket and slowly drenched my messy mop of hair.

"A few specks of rain never hurt anyone!" Morag said. "To the Queen's Head."

We set off back down the long driveway, standing aside to let the stream of black cars pass. The people inside didn't even look at us. It was as though we didn't even exist. At least that way nobody would notice us at the wake either.

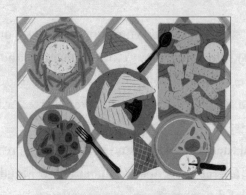

CHAPTER 8

The tips of my fingers were tingly cold by the time we arrived at the Queen's Head. When the vicar said the pub was only down the road, he wasn't lying. But he didn't mention it was a long and busy road, packed with lorries that kept splashing us with muddy puddles.

"I knew I should've brought an umbrella," Morag grumbled as we stepped carefully along a part of the road without a pavement, so we were walking right next to the traffic. "I bet *Imelda* is exactly the type of person to pack a lovely pink spotty umbrella everywhere she goes."

"You don't even own an umbrella," I muttered.

Morag didn't hear what I said over the roar of a

passing bin lorry, which swerved to avoid us. Speckles of dirty road water sprayed our faces as it rushed past.

"Not long now," Morag shouted above the sound of the traffic. "It's only round the corner!"

And then, round the bend in the road, there it was.

The Queen's Head looked posher and bigger than any pub I'd ever seen. It was huge, and had those zigzag castle walls at the top with mini cannons sticking out from between the gaps. The gardens looked fancy and were dotted with metal tables and chairs, not the rotten wooden picnic tables we were used to. There was no way we would blend in here, I thought.

Morag let out a cheer when she saw the pub, punching the air with her gloved fist. She even started dancing in the road, her feet splashing through puddles. She grabbed my hand and dragged me under a concrete bridge towards the pub. I snatched it back and stuffed it deep into my pocket. I hated it when Morag tried to dance with me in public.

"Oh, stop being so miserable, Solo," she said. "We're going to a *party*, for heaven's sake. Lighten up a bit!"

But I felt stiff and tired. I was speckled with mud and dripping with rain. I'd already had enough.

"I want to go home, Morag," I said. My voice came

out more babyish than I wanted. "I'm soaking wet and my shoes keep squelching when I walk."

"Oh, come off it. You'll soon get dry once you're inside. Plus, think of all the amazing food you're about to eat. Don't let a bit of rain spoil your whole life, Solo!"

I wrung out a stream of water from my fringe and it splashed on to the tops of my shoes. This wasn't exactly what I would call a *bit of rain*.

Morag was so soaked that her black eye make-up streamed down her face like a spider reaching out for its prey. Her lacy funeral hat had gone all floppy on her head like a wet flannel. Surely even Morag had to admit that a few free funeral sandwiches weren't worth getting soaking wet, freezing cold and nearly run over for. Maybe it gave her a thrill, sneaking into these places. Not that she would ever admit it.

"Morag, please." I grabbed her hand. "Everyone's going to—"

"Everyone's going to *what*?" she snapped, spinning round, her face so close to mine our noses nearly touched. "We've gone to all this effort, Solo! You want us to go home hungry, is that it?"

"N-no. It's just that I'm really, really cold and I—"

"I'm not just doing this for fun, you know," she hissed. "Don't you think I'd rather be at home with a cuppa? Do you honestly think I enjoy going to all these funerals?"

I went to open my mouth, but I didn't know what to say. Sometimes I *did* think she enjoyed going to the funerals. She seemed to relish the dressing up and meeting people, the getting out and about.

Morag spun on her heels and stormed ahead of me, marching towards the pub through the downpour, her boots clomping on the ground. I don't know why, but my hands actually started shaking then. Stinging tears coated my eyes, but I blinked hard to keep them in.

Sometimes Morag made me want to scream. Part of me wanted to run up and punch her in the back of the leg, to show her how I really felt. But I'd never do that. I'd only feel guilty afterwards; plus, I didn't really want to hurt Morag.

"Well, what about *me*?" I yelled, stamping my foot into a puddle. "What about what *I* enjoy? Why do we never do anything *I* want to do?"

Morag stopped dead, slowly turned on the spot and stared at me as though I'd just called her the worst swear word in the dictionary. I'd really gone and done it.

"I give you everything I can!" she spat. "No one's helping *me*, you know. Your dad's not interested. I've applied for sixteen jobs this month. But, still, I make it work. I put food on the table. Just you try lasting five minutes without me making sure the whole world revolves around you, Solo. Now come on, we're going inside!"

"I'm not going!" I cried, so loud it hurt my throat. "I'm not going in there. We'll only get caught again! Or have you forgotten all about yesterday? You're embarrassing me, Morag!"

I felt guilty as soon as I'd said it. Yes, Morag was embarrassing sometimes, but I still liked her. Sometimes I wished I could press the rewind button on my life and undo the stupid things I said.

"I'm sorry!" I said, moving to follow Morag.

Morag was already halfway across the road, heading for the entrance of the Queen's Head. Before she reached the pavement, she stopped and glared at me.

"You have absolutely no idea what it's like, do you?"

"No idea what *what's* like?" I shouted.

Morag stomped away.

"Morag?"

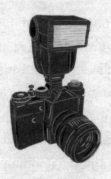

CHAPTER 9

I thought Morag would come and find me if I waited long enough outside in the rain. Turns out I was wrong. I stood there until my fingers were numb and my hair was slicked wet against my head. Sometimes I had to make the first move when it came to making up with Morag.

The Queen's Head pub was so warm my face flushed hot when I stepped through the door. A huge fire made of actual logs crackled in the corner, making everything smell like bonfire smoke. At the other side of the bar was a long, steaming-hot funeral buffet, served on gleaming silver trays. My stomach rumbled and my mouth started to water, but that would have to wait.

I looked this way and that and all around for Morag, but before I had a chance to sweep my sopping fringe out of my face, a bright white flash popped in my face.

I blinked again and again. The bright flash was stuck inside my vision.

"Sorry, guys," a posh-sounding man's voice said, from somewhere in the white light. "You got photo-bombed by the soggy little fella in the suit. I'll have to get another shot. Young man, are you lost? This is a private event."

The man had a camera with a long lens; it hung round his neck on a brown leather strap. A nearby group of grown-ups, all dressed in black, eyeballed me with either disgust or curiosity – I couldn't quite tell. It was only then that I realized he was talking to me.

"Oh, s-sorry," I stuttered. "I'm – I'm just looking for my mum."

"Right. Well, you're in my shot, so…" The photographer gestured for me to get out of the way. "Unless you want to be on the front page of *The Herald* looking like a drowned rat, you might want to skedaddle."

The nearby grown-ups tittered in the same way that the girls at school did when they whispered about me. I shuffled to the side, my feet squelching with every step.

"Much better," the photographer said. "Now, everybody smile – but not too much. It is a funeral, remember. Say cheese! Well, maybe keep your mouths closed, actually."

The flash popped and popped again. The sound was just like a can being crunched under somebody's foot.

I skulked further into the busy pub, cursing those horrible grown-ups for laughing at me. Why did he have to call me a drowned rat? He could've picked a nicer animal – I hated rats and so did everyone else.

But I couldn't waste time thinking about that – I had to find Morag.

I squeezed myself through the gaps between grown-ups dressed in fancy black suits and black fur coats. I ducked beneath designer handbags and smartly dressed waiters carrying silver platters of sparkling drinks and delicious-smelling snacks. Not that they offered me any.

The people here were different from the usual funerals we crashed. Everyone had big hair, white teeth and expensive-looking clothes. They had shiny skin and smelled like the most exotic perfumes. I felt stupid in my sopping charity-shop suit, but luckily most people didn't seem to notice me. People like Morag and me were invisible to people like them.

Morag was proving to be invisible to me too. I walked through every crowded room, and still there was no sign of her. No dripping wet leather jacket, no floppy funeral hat. I even waited outside the ladies' loos for a few minutes, which was really embarrassing. Still no Morag appeared.

Eventually a shrieking, familiar noise soared high over the gentle murmuring of the crowd. It was a cackling laugh that sent chills down my spine. Morag was being loud, and Morag being loud was never a good thing.

I could pick out Morag's laugh anywhere. If somebody blindfolded me and told me to pick out Morag based on her laugh alone, I knew I would nail it one hundred per cent of the time. The sound was exactly like a massive pterodactyl had swooped down and just happened to find everything absolutely hilarious.

Once you'd heard it, everyone remembered Morag's laugh. It was as unique as her fingerprints, and it only belonged to her. I ducked through the moving crowd, following the sound.

Please don't be doing anything embarrassing, I thought. *Please don't be causing a scene.* Sometimes it was as though Morag forgot we hadn't been invited to the funerals. She got too comfortable, made herself at home.

When I finally spotted her, she was leaning against the bar, talking to the young man working behind it. He looked like he wanted to get away from Morag but he was too polite to leave. I knew how he felt. I always wanted to get away from Morag when she started acting all showy-offy.

"Oh, you *are* funny, Alex!" She giggled, tugging on his smart waistcoat. He leaned away from her reach. "You know, I really feel like you and I have a –" she hiccupped – "special connection."

He smiled politely, trying to serve another customer who was waiting patiently, eyeing Morag with curiosity.

"Refill!" Morag shouted, tapping on the side of her empty glass with her long false nails, interrupting. "Come on, don't keep a lady waiting. I'm absolutely parched here!" She cackled as if she'd told the most hilarious joke ever, then looked around to see if anyone else found her as funny as she found herself.

I stepped up beside Morag.

"Here he is!" she yelled, sliding an arm round my shoulder. "My handsome little boy. My *favourite* boy. Sorry about earlier, sweetheart. I've got a lot on my mind today, that's all."

"That's OK," I said. "It doesn't matter."

Morag beckoned to the barman. "Here's my son, the one I told you about! His name is Solo."

"Nice to meet you, Solo," the barman said, giving me a nod. "Think your mum might be enjoying herself a bit too much, don't you?"

"Oh, you flirt!" Morag laughed, swaying a little. "Yes, I enjoy my life. Yes, I like to have – *hic* – fun. Is that a crime? If so, lock me up and throw away the key because I'm – *hic* – guilty as charged, baby!"

Baby? I wanted to projectile-vomit everywhere.

I knew I should try to steer Morag away from the bar, but she was always so stubborn. Whatever I said, Morag would say the opposite. If I wanted chips, Morag wanted a kebab. If I wanted to go home, Morag wanted to stay out all night and watch the sunrise from the top floor of the multi-storey car park in town.

"Can I get you a drink, big man?" Alex the barman was speaking to me. "Lemonade? Coke?"

I went red for some reason. "Lemonade, please," I muttered, looking down at the floor.

"Ooh, look at you ordering your own drinks, Solo. You'll be a professional in no time. You'll be exactly like your old – *hic* – mum."

In one swift move, Morag swiped a handful of miniature cheeseburgers from a passing waiter, almost emptying the entire tray. The waiter looked annoyed but didn't say anything. Morag popped one into her mouth, then slipped the rest into her handbag.

I loved Morag, but I didn't want to be like her when I grew up. She was different from everyone else. What was wrong with just being *normal*? That's what I would be: nice and normal.

Alex gave me my lemonade, and I sucked the sweet liquid into my mouth through the straw until only ice remained. I started shivering as soon as it hit my stomach. Maybe I should have ordered a hot chocolate or a cup of tea, but I didn't know if they did tea in pubs.

"And I'll have the same again." Morag slid her empty glass across the bar. Alex caught it just in time before it smashed on the floor. "Hold the ice. Make it a double."

"Morag," I whispered through clenched teeth. "We're supposed to be getting the food and going straight home, remember? I don't want us to get caught again. We don't even have a proper backstory sorted out."

Morag rolled her eyes. "Can't Mummy have some time to relax with a nice refreshing drink without you being all boring about it?"

Mummy? I never called Morag *Mummy*. She said it made her feel "not like her" whenever anyone called her *Mummy*. As if she'd never had her own life before I came along. She'd always preferred *Morag* ever since I was little. I reckoned she only called herself Mummy when she wanted her own way.

"I didn't think we were staying long," I whined. "I want to go home."

"Fine, fine." Morag picked through her handbag and produced a roll of clear plastic sandwich bags. "Why don't you fill these up to get us started? I'll come and give you a hand after this drink."

I snatched the bags and stuffed them into my pocket. "Fine. Just don't be long."

"Don't forget to have a bite to eat now and all. Might as well make the most of it while we're here."

I took the bags, turned and left without saying anything.

"Solo," Morag whispered, "try not to embarrass us this time, got it?"

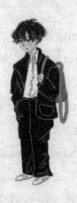

CHAPTER 10

I was a professional at squirrelling away funeral food. My favoured technique was to open up the sandwich bags, placing one inside each of my suit-jacket pockets. There was plenty of space because the pockets were huge, as if they were made for the hands of a giant.

Then I would make my way down the whole length of the buffet, holding a plate. The plate would then become filled to the top with all the elements of the perfect feast. Crispy chicken strips, steak sliders, miniature spring rolls. I always made sure to leave plenty of room for my favourite too: breaded mozzarella dippers.

Once the plate was full, I would find a hidden

corner, away from the crowds. There I would swiftly empty the food into the bags in my pockets and tie a knot at the top of each bag. Of course, I would eat some as well, to make it look realistic that I was there for the funeral. One at a time, the bags would be dropped into Morag's open handbag. Then I'd repeat the process. It was a simple system, but it worked.

"Very good, Solo," she said, after my fourth drop-off. "They've really pulled the stops out for this buffet. Now don't forget to get some of those tempura prawns. You know they're my favourite."

"OK," I grumbled. Morag still wasn't helping. She was more interested in chatting to Alex the barman. As if by magic, her glass kept refilling itself somehow.

"This one will be my last," she purred, leaning over the bar. "Then me and the little one really ought to make a move. Make this one a double, will you?"

"They've all been doubles, darling," Alex the barman sighed, but he made Morag another drink. I was pretty sure it was only fizzy water and ice cubes in the glass this time.

Either way, Morag didn't get a chance to taste it because two big men in black uniforms with crackling walkie-talkies appeared behind her. A reflective strip on their coats read: VENUE SECURITY.

"Excuse me, madam," said the bigger of the two men, tapping Morag's shoulder. "Are you with this young man here?"

Morag turned to face the men. "With him? Well, yeah, he's my son. Oh, don't tell me he's been misbehaving again. What have you gone and done now, Solo?"

"Nothing!" I said, flattening my bulging pockets.

"We've noticed your son's been hanging around that buffet quite a bit. Seems to have quite an appetite on him for such a small fella."

"What exactly are you trying to say?" Morag stood up from her stool and stumbled slightly to the side. "It's a crime to eat food from a buffet now, is it?"

"No, madam, it's not a crime. It's just that we have reason to suspect you weren't invited to this funeral. This is a private event."

"Who do you think you're talking to?" Morag was using her posh voice now. "You ought to – *hic* – mind your lip, you know."

"Now listen, madam. There's no need to be—"

"No need to be *what*?" Morag interrupted. "I'm absolutely – *hic* – fine! Tell them, Solo. Tell them Mummy's fine. I was *invited*! Tell them we were invited!"

I went to open my mouth, but nothing came out. I knew I should stick up for Morag, but I couldn't think of one single word that would make things better.

"Oh, brilliant. Cheers, Solo. Selectively mute as usual. No change there." She turned back to the security guards. "And you two should mind you own – *hic* – business!"

"I'm afraid we're going to have to take a look inside your bag, madam. We trust that won't be an issue."

Morag clutched her handbag close to her stomach. "Absolutely not. There's nothing in there that's any of your business."

The security guards nodded to each other, and in one coordinated movement they hooked their arms under Morag's armpits and lifted her off the stool as if she weighed no more than a feather.

"No!" I cried, my voice returning way too late. "What are you doing? Leave her alone!"

"What on earth are you doing, you – *hic* – brutes?" Morag was screaming at the top of her lungs. "Get your dirty hands off me, you pair of scumbags!"

One of the security guards grabbed Morag's handbag, undid the zipper and held it upside down. Four clear plastic bags filled with funeral food landed on the carpet with a dull thud. Everyone around us gasped in shock, practically sucking all the air from the room.

"I – I've never seen that f-food before in my life!" Morag stuttered. She was pretty good at acting when she needed to. Even I nearly believed her.

I looked at Morag helplessly. What was I meant to do?

"Call the police," one of the security guards told the other. "That's evidence for trespass and theft right there."

"Go on, then – call the police!" Morag snarled. "You'll both be arrested for illegally assaulting a funeral guest! Get off me!"

Finally, I came to life, grabbing Morag's wrist, straining to pull her away from the two guards. They held on to her with what seemed like no effort at all, their grips as strong as iron.

"Just leave her alone!" I screamed. "Let her go!"

"We will, little fella." The security guard smiled annoyingly. "As soon as the police get here!"

I pulled again on Morag's wrist, so hard I felt my veins popping out of my forehead. Why couldn't they just let her go? I wished Morag and I had the power to turn invisible. I wanted us to run away and forget all about this stupid funeral.

That's when the camera flashed. Bright white, right in our faces.

"Oh dear," a man's voice sneered. It was the newspaper photographer from earlier. "What's going on here, then?"

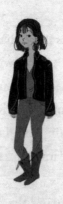

CHAPTER 11

I woke up the next morning to find my damp suit lying crumpled at the bottom of my bed where I'd dumped it last night. The chaos came flooding back like muddy water. My stomach dropped, like when you miss a step on the staircase and you think you might fall right down to the bottom.

So. Embarrassing.

Martin Winner's funeral, the posh black cars, that fancy wake at the Queen's Head. Morag shouting from the middle of the road. Us getting caught with all those bags stuffed with food. That mean photographer from *The Herald*. The blinding light of the camera flash. I pulled the duvet over my head and pushed my face into the pillow. Luckily, the police hadn't arrived in time, so the security guards let us off with a lifetime ban from the Queen's Head.

Getting Morag home had been a nightmare. She wouldn't stop storming off in different directions, babbling to herself. "How *dare* they?" she kept saying. "How *could* they?"

I couldn't stop hearing the sound of those bags of food hitting the carpet. *Thud, thud, thud, thud.* I knew I would be cringing about it for the rest of my life.

The bedroom door creaked open and Morag stepped into the living room, wrapped up in her polka-dot dressing gown.

"Morning, Solo," she croaked, peering at me over the back of the sofa. She looked like a giant from that angle, bearing down from the sky. "Did you manage to sleep all right?"

"I'm OK. How are … you, Morag?" I asked nervously.

"Oh, y'know…" She batted at the air. "Little bit of a headache, but I've had worse. I'll live. I'll be right as rain in a minute."

Did she not remember what happened last night?

"So you haven't got the Big Bad Reds any more?" I asked.

"Don't be silly, Solo," said Morag. "You're always making up stuff to worry about with that imagination of yours. Yes, I was a bit angry with those security guards last night. But that's fine – we'll just make sure we don't go back there for a while."

"For a *while*? Morag, they said we had a lifetime ban!"

"I wouldn't worry about that, Solo. I've had more lifetime bans than you've had hot dinners. Give it a couple of weeks and they'll have totally forgotten about the likes of us."

Morag padded into the kitchen, humming a tune to herself. I couldn't see how the staff at the Queen's Head would ever forget about us. I would remember the look on those security guards' faces for the rest of my life.

The rest of the week passed by in a blur. I just kept my head down at school, trying to keep out of everyone's way, including Miss Carmichael's. I was relieved that there weren't any more funeral parties. I couldn't face another one so soon after the Queen's Head incident.

On Friday morning, I woke up to the sound of Morag in the shower. I heard the water splashing and shampoo being frothed up. She was talking to herself, in between humming along to the radio. Cringing, I realized she was practising for her interview.

"Yes," she said, fake-cheerfully. "I have over eleven years of experience in customer-facing roles. *Oops—*" Then a clatter as something dropped on to the bathtub.

"Oh, absolutely," Morag continued in her imaginary interview. "I thrive when working with the public, particularly when handling complaints or difficult customers."

I rolled my eyes. Morag hated complaints and difficult customers. She called them *posh and entitled pieces of bleep*. Pretty much every day she came home from her job at the train station in a foul mood, ranting and raving about someone being rude to her.

"Ha ha ha!" Morag was laughing at a joke her imaginary interviewer had told. "Certainly. Well, I'm a proven self-starter and I adore taking my own initiative. Equally, I enjoy working as part of a team of colleagues."

The pipes groaned as Morag turned off the shower. She emerged from the bathroom wrapped in her fluffy polka-dot dressing gown, surrounded by a cloud of steam. A nice clean and soapy smell, a mix of strawberries and flowers, drifted out of the bathroom door.

She went to the kitchen and boiled the kettle. "It's interview day. You don't mind coming along, do you? Bit of moral support? It won't take too long, I promise. You can keep yourself busy while I'm in there, can't you?"

"Fine," I said.

I didn't want to go, but it was better than school. Not much happened on Fridays anyway. Still, I hated waiting around for Morag, and there would be nothing fun about waiting outside Bojangles. Knowing my luck, Kai Bailey would find out and tell everyone I was trying on blouses.

Morag went into her bedroom and reappeared holding up two practically identical black tops on hangers. "Which one do you reckon screams Bojangles more?"

I swallowed. I was useless at stuff like that.

Morag didn't talk to me much at the bus stop. She kept doing slow deep breathing and staring at her shaking hands. She wore a black suit, which she had ironed specially, and had paired it with the high-heeled shoes that she saved for best. She actually looked pretty smart.

"The customer is always right," she recited

robotically. "Yes, I'd be more than happy to act as a keyholder. I live less than twenty minutes away."

It was weird seeing Morag so nervous. In everyday life she knew exactly what to say and exactly what to do. But it seemed that job interviews made Morag go blank, so she had to practise loads before. That's why I always got dragged along as Morag's lucky charm. Something about me being there helped Morag remember her words, apparently.

The plan was always the same when we arrived. I had to separate from Morag before she got to the door, so that they didn't know she had a son. Some jobs didn't like that, for some reason. Then I was to wait outside in a hidden location for as long as it took her to reappear. I could always tell whether it had gone badly just from the look on Morag's face. Recently they had always gone badly.

"How do I look?" She twirled round.

"Awesome. Very smart."

"Done up or undone?" she asked, buttoning her jacket, then undoing it. It didn't make any difference, so I just shrugged.

"Do you think you'll get this one, Morag?"

"Fingers, toes and eyeballs crossed," she said. "If I get this, we can stop doing the funerals, which would be nice. Maybe I can even save up for a trip to Sunset Dunes this summer."

"That would be so awesome." I could practically taste the slushies, salty chips and sea air. I loved Sunset Dunes. I wanted to go back so much that I crossed my fingers in my pockets.

"We'll have to hope they're not too stuffy," Morag said. "I might have to put on a few airs and graces."

"You'll be fine. You said they were nice on the phone!" I held up my palm for a high-five, excited for our holiday. Morag patted it weakly, which was kind of a downer.

"I hate it," she muttered. "I hate having to pretend to be someone I'm not to get a job. I'm perfectly capable of folding some clothes and putting them in a bag. I don't see why I have to pretend to be some sort of brain surgeon."

I had no idea what to say. I'd never been to an interview, and I wasn't sure I liked the sound of them. People asking difficult questions and judging your answers. It sounded too much like a lesson with Miss Cowmichael.

"Then half the time they say they've found somebody more passionate," Morag went on. "That's what they said at that warehouse before. How *passionate* do they want me to be about packing boxes with individual pouches of cat food?"

Then Morag stuck her hand out into the road. Our bus screeched to a halt as if it hadn't seen us. It looked busy, with people pressed up against the windows and doors.

Morag tutted. "That's all I need. Packed in like sardines. Come on, Solo. Stay close. We don't have time to wait for the next one."

We stood by the driver, waiting for a space to clear between the passengers.

"Come on, come on," Morag grumbled, jittering.

"Excuse me, are you Morag Walker?" a voice said.

We both spun round. A man who I'd never seen before was standing behind us on the pavement, looking as though he was boarding the bus.

"Why? Who's asking?" Morag said.

The man said nothing. He held a camera up to his eye and a bright flash popped, just like it had the other night. The doors closed, and we watched him as the bus pulled away.

"What on earth was that all about?" Morag muttered. "Absolute weirdo."

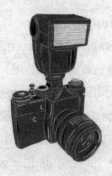

CHAPTER 12

"There it is," Morag said. She had got more nervous after that strange man took our photo. She kept rehearsing her lines under her breath and messing them up. "Bojangles boutique. Looks quite nice, doesn't it?"

It did look nice. The Bojangles sign above the door was done in a gold handwriting style, and the clothes in the window looked like clothes that people wore to award shows on telly. A woman with long blonde hair appeared in the window and draped a silky scarf round the shoulders of one of the mannequins.

"That could be me," Morag said. "I reckon I could do that, don't you? Maybe I'll suggest a nice leather jacket for the other mannequin. They'll like that.

89

Showing a bit of initiative."

"Go for it, Morag," I said, trying to sound excited. "Show them what you're made of!"

"Yeah." She nodded. "Yeah, positive mindset and all. What's the worst that can happen, eh?"

Morag looked at her watch and started to pace in circles. She shook her hands like when we did cooldown at the end of PE. It got the tension out of our bodies, apparently. It didn't seem to be working too well for Morag.

"Just be yourself," I said. "And don't forget to smile."

Morag smiled a little too much and gave me two thumbs up. "Don't go wandering off. I'll be back out in half an hour. Wish me luck!"

"Good luck!"

I sat on a bench and watched Morag crossing the road. There was a kind of confidence in her walk that made her look even smarter in her suit, like someone powerful. I shoved both hands into my pockets and crossed all my crossable fingers. This interview had to go well.

On the opposite pavement, a woman was running behind Morag, trying to catch up with her. I thought perhaps Morag had dropped something, her phone maybe. Then I saw the microphone in the woman's hand. Behind her was a man struggling with a heavy camera that rested on his shoulder.

Morag had just pushed open the door to Bojangles when the woman reached her and shoved the microphone right in front of Morag's face. Morag looked shocked, then confused. Then she started shaking her head. She said something to the woman and pushed the microphone away.

"Morag! What's going on?" I shouted, but she couldn't hear me because of the traffic. It looked like they were arguing. I tried to read their lips, but a bus blocked my view.

I ran round the bus, just in time to see Morag turning to the cameraman and shoving the long lens away, sending the man stumbling backwards. She was shouting now, her finger pointing into the man's face. The woman kept shouting after Morag as the door of Bojangles slammed shut.

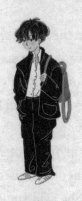

CHAPTER 13

It didn't take long for Morag to reappear from Bojangles, followed by the blonde lady we'd spotted in the window. The lady stood with her arms folded, scowling at Morag, who stormed across the road, red in the face.

"How did it go?" I asked, even though I knew it wasn't good news.

"Come on – we're leaving." Morag grabbed my sleeve and tugged me along with her. "Absolute waste of time."

"What happened? Who were those people?" I was running to keep up with Morag's extra-long strides. "What did that woman with the microphone say to you? Are you going to be on telly?"

"It doesn't matter." Her voice sounded strange and tight. She was walking so fast that people were turning to watch.

"Did you get the job?"

"Don't be silly," she spat. "Apparently my behaviour outside didn't represent Bojangles' core values and clientele. Didn't want to work there anyway. *Bojangles*. Stupid name for a shop if you ask me. Probably shouldn't have told her that, mind."

"Why are people trying to take pictures of you?"

"Stop it, Solo. I've had enough of your questions!"

I followed Morag as she marched into a corner shop, crashing past the vegetables and sweets and packets of crisps. A giant display of magazines and newspapers covered the far wall. She started rummaging through them at speed.

Finally, she found some copies of *The Herald*. The colour drained from Morag's face as she took in the front page.

DRUNK MUM CRASHES
FOOTBALL LEGEND MEMORIAL

Beneath it was a large black-and-white photo of a woman surrounded by two big security guards in black uniforms. In front of her was an empty handbag and four plastic bags filled with food. In the corner of the picture was a boy shouting and trying to prise the guards' hands off the woman.

The woman was Morag. The boy was me.

That's when everything changed for ever.

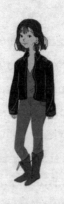

CHAPTER 14

"*No, no, no.*" Morag bashed her hand against the kitchen table three times. *Bang. Bang. Bang.* The sound of her voice was muffled by her arms. "Tell me this isn't happening, Solo. Tell me this isn't happening!"

She'd been saying that over and over again since we got home. I didn't know what to do. It was like I couldn't speak. My ears were ringing. I felt dizzy and sick.

I walked back to the table and picked up the newspaper again. It was real. My hands shook so much I could barely hold it. The thin pages were trembling and the corners kept rolling inwards and getting in the way.

The Herald can exclusively report that a brazen single mum will stop at nothing for a free meal and a few drinks on the house. Morag Walker of Elmstow Court Flats in south London was caught red-handed filling empty bags and lunchboxes with food at the wake of a football legend on Monday night. Ms Walker has a history of funeral crashing, and countless locals have come forward with similar stories.

I felt a tremble deep down in my stomach, and not the hungry kind. How did they know Morag's name? How did they know our address? Did that mean they knew my name too?

Morag had a weird, blank expression on her face. Her cheeks were tear-stained and she'd gone a funny colour, like a mixture between green and white.

"My whole life is ruined," she muttered. "It's all totally ruined."

I didn't know what to say, so I just kept reading.

Ms Walker, aged 38, lives with her ten-year-old son, Solo, whom she regularly brings along to funerals and wakes as a distraction to prevent other guests from noticing their ongoing scam...

I felt sick. What if Dad saw the article? He'd probably be happy to see Morag getting in trouble. He might even try to take me away from Morag. The last thing I wanted, though, was him or Evil Imelda to start bossing me about and pretending like they cared about me.

The greedy Ms Walker's shameless ploy came to a dramatic conclusion when she was forcibly removed from the wake of football legend Martin Winner, after downing countless free drinks and filling plastic bags with food.

A security attendant at the Queen's Head pub was quoted as saying: "An uninvited funeral crasher was indeed removed from a private event this evening. We take any invasion of our guests' privacy very seriously...

Members of the public planning to hold a funeral, wake or memorial service are being warned to remain vigilant for uninvited scammers who might be hoping to invade your loved one's special day.

"Morag?" I said. "What're scammers?"

"I told you – don't ask silly questions, Solo," she

snapped, her head twisting round like a dragon woken from its slumber.

I walked over and put a hand on her shoulder, but she jerked away as though my hand was a boiling-hot poker.

"*GET OFF ME, SOLO! JUST LEAVE ME ALONE!*"

I flinched and stumbled backwards.

"Don't you understand?" Morag groaned. "Everyone knows now. Absolutely everyone."

She opened the bag from the corner shop and pulled out a glass bottle filled with brownish liquid. The label said PREMIUM SCOTTISH WHISKY – SUPER GREAT VALUE! I had never tried Premium Scottish Whisky, but I knew it meant trouble for Morag.

She got up and headed to her bedroom.

"But, Morag, where do you expect me to go—"

"*JUST GO! ANYWHERE JUST GO, GO, GO AWAY!*"

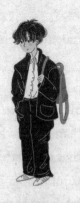

CHAPTER 15

SPLAT.

I opened my eyes. Another grey Monday.

I'd been having the most brilliant dream about me, Dad and Morag. In the dream we lived in America in a massive posh house with a gleaming blue swimming pool in the back garden. I even had my own puppy called Lucky. We realized that Disney World was right at the bottom of our garden, so we all went down to—

SPLAT.

I turned to the window. Something white and very gooey was trickling down the outside of the glass. It looked like a bird had done a massive poo all over it. But the only bird that could do a poo that

99

big would be colossal, and there weren't any colossal birds around here.

SPLAT.

And again! Now there were orange bits in it too, and hard bits, smearing the glass in a horrible, congealed mess. What on earth was going on?

SPLAT, SPLAT.

I pushed my duvet down to my feet. There was sleep in the corner of my eyes, and my head felt all foggy. I squinted to look closer at the mess. White, orange, bits of shell. Eggshell.

Somebody was throwing eggs at our window!

SPLAT, SPLAT, SPLAT.

I bolted up and out of bed in my pyjamas, feeling the chilly air wrap my bare ankles. When I reached the window, I flung it open as wide as I could. An egg flew through the gap, missing my head by a scratch. It splatted all across the sofa in a horrible mess.

"Nice one, Kai!" I heard someone shout. "You nearly got him right in the head!"

"What are you doing?" I screamed, leaning out of the window. "Stop it! You're ruining our windows!"

There were about six boys on bikes in the car park outside our block of flats. Each boy was armed with a box of six eggs. They all laughed and started mimicking me.

"*You're ruining our windows!*" one of the boys whined back at me in a baby voice. "What are you going to do? Call security?"

Most of them were older boys who were wearing the uniform from the Big School. But I recognized one of the scrawny, mean faces immediately. It was Kai Bailey. Kai Bailey from my class.

"Shouldn't you be at a funeral?" one of them hollered, their voice echoing around the neighbourhood. "Stealing dead people's sandwiches?"

They all cackled like a group of stupid hyenas.

"Just go away!" I yelled. "Go away or else!"

"Or what? Are you going to come out and stop us?"

"He's probably too busy chasing coffins to chase after us!"

Then they all started chanting in unison: "*Funeral boy! Funeral boy! Funeral boy! Funeral boy!*"

Great, I thought. *Another nickname to add to the list.* Right after weirdo, freak, Hands Solo and Walker's Crisps. *Funeral Boy. Please don't let this one stick*, I pleaded to no one in particular.

"Go away, or I'll have to get Morag on to you!" I bellowed. "You won't know what's hit you then!"

"Whatever, funeral freak!" Kai shouted. "Your mum lays one finger on us and she'll get taken to prison and you'll have to go and live in a children's home for ever!"

They all started cheering and laughing again. Our nosy neighbours were watching from their windows, lurking behind their net curtains. Grumpy Mr Thurston from across the hall would freak out when he saw the mess.

"Yeah, well, you'll be in hospital by the time Morag's done with you!" I shouted back.

"Aww, you sound cranky, Funeral Boy! Is Funeral Boy hungry? Sounds like you and *Mummykins* up there fancy another omelette!"

"*FIRE!*"

I slammed the window so hard that the whole block shuddered. A split second later, a whole flock of flying eggs smashed against the glass like bullets from a machine gun.

SPLAT, SPLAT, SPLAT, SPLAT, SPLAT.

I pulled the curtains closed, plunging the living room into darkness. I couldn't let Morag see the mess or she would hit the roof. She hadn't got out of bed since she read the article in the paper. Hopefully the rain would come soon and wash all the eggs away.

SPLAT, SPLAT, SPLAT.

I fetched a tea towel from the kitchen and started wiping the egg off the sofa, my hands shaking. I hated those boys so much. Especially Kai Bailey.

I closed my eyes and imagined me turning up to school one day with muscles so huge that Kai would cower away in tears after just one look at me. He would be so scared he would wet his pants on the spot in front of everyone in the whole school, and he'd have to wear a pair of horrible flowery girls' shorts from Lost Property for the rest of his life.

"What the hell's going on, Solo? What's all the racket about?"

My daydream fell apart around me like a house collapsing in on itself. I hid the tea towel and pieces of eggshell behind my back.

Morag was standing outside her open bedroom door, rubbing her eyes. Her hair stuck out at weird angles, and her eyes looked blurry and smudged. I'd taken her cups of tea and biscuits all day yesterday, but I could see she hadn't touched them. The tea had grown a whiteish skin on top.

"It's nothing!" I grinned, hoping she wouldn't walk over and open the curtains. "Some stupid boys playing tricks outside, that's all."

SPLAT, SPLAT, SPLAT.

I clenched my jaw. Why weren't they stopping?

But Morag didn't say anything. She just stared at the floor.

"Are you all right, Morag? Do you need some breakfast? I can do toast."

"You should get ready for school," she said, ignoring my question. Fear twisted in my chest. Kai Bailey would be at school. Melissa's mean girl gang would be there too. They'd all have seen the papers.

"No!" I protested. "I can't go!" I ran over and wrapped my arms round her waist. "Please say you won't make me go!"

"*Get. Off. Meeee,*" she grumbled as she freed herself, prising me off.

She shuffled back to her bedroom and slammed the door. I heard the sound of her mattress squeaking as she got back into bed.

"Morag?" I said through the closed door. "Did you manage to get my uniform? ... Morag?"

There was no response.

I felt sick while I was putting the eggshell pieces in the bin, but it wasn't just the stink. It was the thought of school.

Maybe I was making things worse in my head, like Morag always said.

Kai might not have told anybody. Maybe I could convince him to keep quiet. Plus, nobody reads newspapers any more, right?

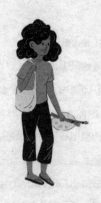

CHAPTER 16

Wrong.

"Solo! Wait up, Solo!"

I turned to see Miss Ellis the teaching assistant running across the playground towards me. She worked in class for art and music. Her brown curly hair bounced as she ran.

"Solo, wait for me!"

I tried to carry on walking. I wasn't in the mood to talk, but she caught up to me in no time, and it felt too rude to properly ignore her. After all, Miss Ellis was one of the nice ones.

"Do you have two seconds, Solo? I know you're running a bit late, but I'll tell Miss Carmichael it was my fault – not to worry."

"What is it?" I asked.

"Listen, I…" Miss Ellis shifted her weight awkwardly from one sandal to another. "I saw something in the news about you and your mum. About the funeral… I suppose I just wanted to check in and ask whether you're all right."

"Oh, that." I stared at the ground.

"Yeah, that," she said quietly. "Can't be nice having your business splashed all over the papers. If you need anyone to talk to, you know where I am, OK?"

"Sure," I said. I wanted to be anywhere else but here, having this conversation. "I really should go to class now."

"How about your mum? Is she doing all right?"

"She's fine," I said, my voice sounding all raspy and weird.

Miss Ellis started rummaging in her handbag. "Listen, I have something to give you. It's information about a local food bank. Do you know what that is, Solo?"

I shrugged, but of course I'd heard of them. Sometimes school sent a letter home asking for donations of food and other bits for the local food bank. Back when Morag had her job, she used to send me in with tins and pasta and washing-up liquid for the collection. It wasn't much, just things she didn't need. I hadn't dared suggest to Morag that maybe we could go to the food bank. Morag hated when people tried to help her.

"It's a local organization designed to help people in difficult situations," Miss Ellis went on. "I volunteer there a few times a week and everyone is super nice and totally non-judgemental. They can help you out with food and essentials if you and your mum need it. And it's all totally free of charge."

She handed me a leaflet with a smaller piece of paper inside that said FOOD BANK VOUCHER at the top. Underneath the heading, there was an address, a phone number and different blank sections to be filled in.

"Show it to your mum. All she needs to do is add a bit of information, bring it to the centre, and we'll do the rest."

"Thanks," I said, and I folded them up and stuffed them inside my jacket pocket. I didn't know whether I dared show Morag. "I'd better be going."

"And, Solo…" Miss Ellis looked me in the eye and sounded serious. "I won't tell anyone about what we've spoken about this morning. There's no need to worry about that."

That was something, I supposed.

Miss Carmichael was halfway through the register when I got to the classroom door. It was open, but I stood there for ages, unsure whether to go in. Sometimes Miss Carmichael didn't mind people being late. Other times she pretty much bit the latecomer's head clean off, like a carnivorous beast.

"Katy McDonald?" I heard her call out.

"Yes, Miss Carmichael."

"Morning, Katy. Nathaniel Neville?"

"Yes, Miss Carmichael."

"Good morning, Nathaniel. Nice haircut, by the way. Sebastian Olivers?"

"Yes, Miss Carmichael. And, Miss? There's *somebody* waiting at the door, Miss."

Miss Carmichael turned and saw me, then the whole class started giggling. I didn't move.

"Ah, Solo Walker," she said, not sounding happy. She popped the lid back on her pen. "Better late than never. Are you coming in?"

I swallowed. "Yes, Miss Carmichael. Sorry I'm late. I—"

"Yes? And what's the reason today?"

I felt Miss Cowmichael's eyes glaring right through

me, reading my thoughts, inspecting the piece of toast I had for breakfast. I hadn't even bothered to make up an excuse while I was running to school. I opened my mouth to speak but only a croak came out.

"He was probably at a funeral, Miss!" somebody shouted.

"Oh dear," she said. "I'm sorry for your loss, Solo."

Everyone immediately burst out laughing and I felt my face start to inflate like a balloon at a birthday party.

So they knew. Great.

"Yeah, he was probably too busy having *eggs* for breakfast," said Kai Bailey, looking smug. All the boys on Kai's table could barely contain their smirks. He'd obviously told them what he'd done to our windows.

"I haven't been to a funeral, Miss," I croaked.

"What's all this nonsense about, then?" she said, indicating Kai and his mates.

"It's nothing," I said. "Just a stupid joke, that's all."

"Well, that's enough joking around. Now, you know what I'm going to say, don't you, Solo?" Miss Carmichael glanced at my clothes. "I'm afraid it's going to be another demerit for uniform."

Everybody laughed again.

"That's just one more demerit before I'll have to

send a letter home, OK. We're having a uniform sale next week, as it happens," she continued. "All right, Solo, you can take your seat while I finish the register."

"Yes, Miss Carmichael."

I made my way to my usual table, muttering a curse at Kai under my breath as I scuffed my shoes along the carpet. I knew I didn't really have magical powers, but it was always worth a shot.

When I got to my seat, someone was already sitting in it. Someone I'd never seen before in my life, right there in my chair. She had long, shiny black hair and a uniform so neat and tidy it had straight lines ironed down the sleeves. She was even wearing the gleaming gold Star of the Week pin badge.

"Sorry." The girl shrugged. "I think this seat's mine now. I'm new."

"New?" I said.

"Yeah," said Mina, sucking on the end of her pink pen. "Chetna sits on this table now. We actually call it the *Cool Table* since *you* don't sit here any more. Don't we, Chetna?"

Chetna shrugged again.

"What? When did you start?" I looked around in disbelief.

"I started on Friday. You weren't here, so Miss

Carmichael told me to—"

"But you're already Star of the Week!" I said. "How did you even get it?"

"That's none of your beeswax, FB." Mina flicked her hair, creating a curtain between her and me.

FB? I thought. *Oh. Funeral Boy.*

"Ah, yes." Miss Carmichael appeared and ushered me along. "Chetna is a new student in the class. You'll have to take a chair and work on your lap for the time being. I'll ask Mr Stephens the caretaker to bring in another desk after lunch."

Everyone watched me as I lifted a chair from the stack in the corner and sat down on my own in the space next to the fire exit.

"Long division, what joy!" Miss Carmichael announced, which wasn't funny, but everyone chuckled. "We'll be picking up exactly where we left off in last week's lesson."

She began scrawling numbers and lines all over the whiteboard. Instantly I was lost, like the time I wandered off at the supermarket and ended up in the freezer section looking at ice cream. Meanwhile Morag had been panicking in the vegetable aisle. That was years ago. Nowadays it was me who went looking for her.

My eyes started to go blurry. I got my jotter out of my school bag and drew a massive robot called Solobot 3000 on the back page. It had a square metal head, pointy fangs, four guns coming out of each hand, and huge crusher feet the size of double-decker buses. I drew Kai Bailey underneath one of the feet, with crosses for his eyes to show he was a goner.

I glanced up and noticed that Chetna wasn't facing the board. She had turned round in her seat (well, my seat, technically) and she was looking directly at *me*.

What? I mouthed, making my eyes all small and mean. I already knew I was going to be called Funeral Boy for ever; I didn't need the new girl to remind me.

But rather than sticking out her tongue or saying something cruel, the girl did the strangest thing. She smiled.

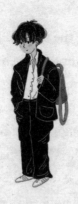

CHAPTER 17

That lunchtime was the worst lunchtime ever. Fish pie for mains, served with peas and potato smilies that were so burnt they looked really upset. Dessert was tinned fruit and yoghurt, which, as far as I'm concerned, ought to be illegal.

Kai made things worse when he shouted, "These potato smilies are practically cremated. Solo would know!" Then everyone laughed because he's *so* hilarious.

The only person who didn't laugh was Chetna, but I wasn't sure why. The Cool Table were hogging her and showing off because she was new.

I tried flicking some peas at Kai with my spoon in retaliation but got told off by a dinner lady before I had a chance to release the ammo. Luckily, dinner ladies can't give demerits or I would have been done for.

After we ate, I retreated to one of my lunchtime hiding places, under the stairs by the changing rooms. Since last week though, it had been filled with a huge stinky pile of cracked gym mats. I tried to squeeze myself into a crevice down the side of the pile, but I couldn't fit.

So instead I slunk around the silent corridors while everyone else played outside. I could hear the *boom*, *boom*, *boom* of footballs being kicked against walls, echoing like thunder in the empty halls.

Eventually I found myself alone in the cloakroom with everyone's backpacks and abandoned coats. It was gross in the cloakroom. The floor was sticky, and the air smelled like old packed lunches and lost property.

I pinched my nose as I walked past smelly PE kit bags. When I reached the hooks at the very end, I parted the hanging coats and bags and made myself a nest, where I hid, imagining I was a hibernating dormouse inside its hole.

I liked my hiding place beneath the coats. The fleecy linings of the coats were soft and fluffy. I could tell that these kids' parents used fancy fabric softener.

They smelled of flowers and sweets and fresh country air. It started to get warmer and warmer in my coat nest, and I started to feel like I was in my alcove behind the sofa, getting ready for some really good dreams.

Thinking about home reminded me of Morag. I wondered whether she would still be feeling upset, or whether she would be acting cheery and nice and put cartoons on for me. That was the trouble with Morag. You never knew which version you were going to get.

I nearly drifted off. In fact, I must have done, because the bell rang and made me jump like an electric current running through me. I'd missed all of lunch break. Mission accomplished.

Everyone started running into the cloakroom, some dumping skipping ropes and footballs in their backpacks, but nobody discovered me tucked away under all the coats.

It was strange, crouching there, out of sight. I listened to them talking about the games they'd played outside and about someone who'd fallen over and grazed their knee on the concrete. Not one person knew I was right there, hidden in a nest made of their very own coats.

Well, that was until Melissa Underwood decided to take her coat off the hook. I think her coat was the one that smelled sort of good, like a field of fresh daisies. The coat lifted and I closed my eyes as the bright light poured into my nest. I thought about running away, but I knew it was too late. I'd been caught.

When she saw me, Melissa just stood there, staring at me for like ten seconds. I stared back, noticing her blonde pigtails and pink lip gloss that she was always going on about. Then she let out a piercing scream as if she'd stumbled upon a hideous creature.

Her friends – Stacey, Missy, Ameyo and Mina – all started screaming too, shouting "Gross!" and "What is Funeral Boy *doing* under there?" and "Why is he such a *weirdo*?"

"Why were you sniffing my coat, you total complete *oddball*?" Melissa shrieked.

"S-sorry," I stuttered. "I didn't know it was your coat. I was only hiding—"

"Do you *fancy* Melissa, is that it?" Ameyo sneered. "Because, news flash, she's totally, one hundred per cent out of your league."

The girls stood there, their eyes moving up and down from my hair to my shoes. They reminded me of the mean girls I'd seen on American telly shows.

"I don't fancy her!" I said.

I absolutely did *not* fancy Melissa Underwood. In fact, I thought she was the worst girl in the whole school. She was a massive teacher's pet, always kissing up to Miss Cowmichael and constantly trying to get Star of the Week.

"So you're saying Melissa's ugly now, are you?" Mina chipped in. "You should thank your lucky stars she's even willing to talk to a scrub like you. Because let me tell you one thing, Melissa is the prettiest girl in this whole school, got it?"

"But I never said that!"

"*Miss Carmichael! Miss Carmichael!*" Melissa shrieked. "Solo's being weird again!"

"What's going on in here, girls?" a grown-up's voice said. Miss Ellis had appeared round the corner. I was starting to think she was following me. "What's all the fuss about?"

"Solo was hiding under our coats!" Melissa yelled.

"Yeah, he was *smelling* them," Mina added.

"Oh dear," said Miss Ellis. "I'm sure it's all just a misunderstanding, don't you think?"

"He was, Miss! He was really inhaling it!"

"He's a coat-sniffing freak," Ameyo said. "He clearly fancies Melissa – that's why he chose her coat."

"Ameyo," Miss Ellis said. She came over and looked down at me, still crouching among the scattered coats. "We try not to use hurtful language, don't we? That'll be a demerit for you."

"But, Miss Ellis!" the girls protested in unison.

"We don't use that language," she repeated more firmly. "I'll have a chat with Solo. Now, back to class, all of you."

The girls filed away to Miss Carmichael's classroom, leaving me there with Miss Ellis. I wanted to disappear.

"I was only hiding," I muttered.

Miss Ellis bent down till her eyes were level with mine. "Hiding from what?"

I shrugged. "I don't know. Everything."

Miss Ellis nodded slowly. "It must be tough. We all want to hide sometimes. Don't let narrow-minded people bring you down, Solo," she said with a smile. Then she straightened up, turned and walked away, her lanyard jangling. "I'll see you for art in a few minutes. Don't be late!"

"OK."

"Chop, chop, Solo, we're starting our collages!" Miss Cowmichael said, as I walked through the door.

Miss Ellis was standing next to Miss Cowmichael. She gave me a knowing wink.

"Sorry, Miss Carmichael. I must have lost track of the time."

"*He was probably asleep in a coffin*," somebody muttered. A burst of laughter erupted.

Miss Carmichael clapped her hands three times. "Come on, class. That's enough talking – it's concentration time."

I tiptoed back to my chair at the back of the room. Everyone eyeballed me like I was a green alien with seven heads or something, rather than a boy arriving five minutes late from lunch. Ameyo and Melissa glared at me particularly fiercely.

Don't let narrow-minded people bring you down. I repeated it over and over again.

"Luckily for us, we have the lovely Miss Ellis here helping us this afternoon," Miss Carmichael announced. "We'll be producing nature collages for the classroom display. First, let's get into groups of your choice and start to plan your collages."

My heart sank all the way down to the soles of my feet. Three words I hated: *get into groups*. No one ever wanted to work with me. I was always the last one to be picked for anything, from football to French verbs, without fail. Now that I was table-less, Miss Cowmichael would have to stick me on to someone else's group like an unnecessary wheel on a bike.

"We've got paper, pens and scissors at the front of the class. The theme is nature. Think about the seasons. Think about wildlife you've seen in the local area. Your collage should reflect your favourite things about the natural world!" Miss Cowmichael went on. "No paint on the tables please. I'll be counting the glitter markers at the end. We don't want them sneaking home in anybody's pencil cases, so no one goes home until all fifteen are returned, got it?"

I sat still while everyone hurried to get paper and pens and scissors, before gathering in their groups.

Why was it always me with no partner? I wished I could click my fingers and disappear into thin air. Trouble was, Morag hadn't taught me how to click my fingers yet.

"Do you not have a partner, Solo?" Miss Ellis was standing in front of me, smiling.

I shook my head. I hoped she wasn't going to try to make me pair up with her, which would be even more embarrassing than working alone.

"That's OK," she said. "Chetna, are you looking for a group?"

"Yes, I am, as it happens," Chetna said confidently.

"What do you say, Solo?" said Miss Ellis.

I shrugged and looked at the floor. Chetna's school shoes were so shiny and new I could see my reflection staring back at me.

"OK," I mumbled.

"Good," said Miss Ellis before turning away. "Perhaps we can borrow a desk from over here…"

"Is this some sort of trick?" I said to Chetna as she came over to sit next to me. "Are you pretending to want to work with me so you can laugh about me with the Cool Table?"

"No," she said. "I'm not playing tricks, pinky swear!" She held her little finger out towards me like a curled-up prawn from my favourite dish at Noodle Town – it was where me and Morag used to go before things changed.

"What's a pinky swear? It's not like that wet-finger thing Kai always does, is it?" I'd had enough of Kai's spit-soaked fingers stuffed into my ears to last a lifetime. Wiping my ear with my shoulder, I shuddered away the memory.

"It just means *I promise*, that's all. I saw it on TV."

"Oh." I'd never seen a pinky swear on TV. "What do I do?"

"Just link your little pinky finger with mine and shake it around a bit."

"Like this?" I curled my little finger round hers and shook it like we were rattling an unbreakable chain.

Chetna smiled. "There you go. Now we're a fully fledged collage team!"

"Wouldn't you rather be in a team with Mina and the rest of the Cool Table gang?" I asked.

Chetna screwed her nose up. "Mina says I need to get scented glitter gel pens and a new pencil case if I want to be considered a core member of the Cool Table."

"Maybe you can ask your mum and dad to buy you them. Then they'll let you in, I'm sure."

"Maybe I just don't care *that* much about scented pens." Chetna smiled secretly, her back to the Cool Table. "It's what you write with them that's important."

I hid my notebook behind my back, hoping that Chetna wouldn't notice that my handwriting looked like a family of half-squashed spiders scuttling across the page.

I wasn't sure why she was being so nice. Didn't Chetna know about me and Morag being in the news for crashing funerals? Clearly she didn't.

"Right, then. I'll get the coloured paper. You can go and find some scissors sharp enough to cut it up, OK? Not the left-handed ones, please. And a glue stick! Then you really need to tell me why on *earth* you're called Funeral Boy."

Great.

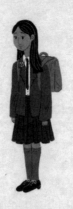

CHAPTER 18

I ran home from school like a character in a movie with big, big news to share. It had been the weirdest day. First the egg-splatting, then Miss Ellis giving me the information about the food bank, then Miss Cowmichael and the demerit, then me hiding under the coats and Miss Ellis sticking up for me. Then Chetna came along and changed *everything*.

Chetna was so smart. It was her idea to print out actual photos of foxes, badgers, woodpeckers and squirrels using the computer to make our collage into a forest. Ours was the only one with *real* photos. Everyone else's had bad drawings that looked babyish. Chetna wrote true facts about the animals in smart handwriting, like: *Grey squirrels are not native to the*

United Kingdom. Miss Carmichael loved our collage so much she put it on the wall there and then, right in the middle of the display.

Sure, Chetna did most of the work, but she told me I was good at cutting out the leaf shapes and particularly skilled with the glue. It was strange how things could change so quickly.

Best of all, I told Chetna about the whole Funeral Boy thing and she didn't even care. I couldn't believe it. She said she'd rather do a collage with a funeral-crasher than a member of the Cool Table or any of Kai's cronies.

Chetna told me that, in some cultures, people go along to funerals even if they didn't know the person that died. She said it was something to do with community and traditions. I couldn't wait to tell Morag all about that. Maybe it would cheer her up a bit.

My footsteps echoed as I ran up the stairs to the flat, taking them two at a time, rushing past the growing mountain of unopened letters, bills and rent reminders on the shared post table.

"Morag!" I pushed through the front door and stumbled into the hallway, dropping my backpack and suit jacket by the door. "Morag! Where are you? I've got so much to tell you, Morag!"

"In here," came the croaked reply.

I stepped into the living room. All the lights were off and the flat was cold. Morag was curled up in front of the paused TV. She still looked pretty depressed. The egg on the windows had dried into a yellowy-white crust.

"You won't believe what's happened today, Morag! First everything *was* a bit rubbish, but then there was this new girl called Chetna, and we did this collage of a forest and Miss Carmichael said it was the best one out of the whole class!"

"Sounds lovely," said Morag. Her voice was all quiet and weird, like when I'd done something wrong and really upset her.

"Chetna only started at our school last week. Chetna printed off loads of photos and wrote facts about all the animals on our collage. Chetna has the best handwriting I've literally ever seen."

Morag didn't reply. She just stared blankly at the paused TV. The picture flickered as though it was itching to move and couldn't stay stopped.

"Is something the matter, Morag?"

"What do you think?" she said. "Only my whole miserable life being splashed all over the newspapers for everyone to see, that's all."

I slid gently on to the sofa beside her. "Yeah, but Chetna said that in some cultures—"

"Oh, Chetna, Chetna, Chetna!" Morag snapped. "I've never heard of this girl in my whole life, now she's all you're going on about!"

"Sorry, Morag." I needed to change the subject. "Melissa and Ameyo were mean. Mina called me a scrub, and Ameyo said I fancied Melissa, but Melissa's *annoying* and *mean* and I'd *never* fancy her—"

Morag chuckled flatly. "Mina used to eat handfuls of play dough when you were at nursery together. Handfuls and handfuls of it, honestly. She isn't all that, Solo. Even if she makes out she is."

I paused, picturing Mina shovelling fistfuls of colourful play dough into her gob.

Morag grinned. "She must've liked the taste or something. Her mum used to have to get it out from between her teeth with floss. She told me about it at pick-up time."

I burst out laughing then.

Morag still seemed flat though. She kept staring into space and shaking her head as if answering a question that nobody was asking.

"Miss Ellis gave me this." I handed the crumpled food-bank leaflet and voucher to Morag. "She said there's a place we can get free food instead of the funerals. They're nice, apparently."

She took the papers, raised her eyebrows and then tossed the sheets to the side. "Tell her thanks but we won't be needing it."

"But, Morag—"

"Enough, Solo," she snapped. "I don't want other people saying I can't cope, OK? I'm coping *perfectly fine*."

"Fine," I grumbled. I sat next to Morag and stared at the carpet.

"Chetna said in some cultures people actually go to the funerals of people they don't even know," I said, feeling braver. "So what we did wasn't even that bad. It happens all the time, all over the world."

Morag started laughing, and I knew everything was OK. Chetna was right; it wasn't a big deal. Now Morag and I could go back to normal. I smiled, proud of myself for fixing Morag's Big Bad Reds.

But Morag didn't stop laughing. She laughed and laughed for ages, until I started to think maybe she was actually crying.

"What's the matter, Morag?"

She pressed a button on the remote and the telly came to life. Five posh ladies with white teeth and nice clothes were sitting around a desk. The audience clapped and cheered as they returned from the advert break.

"Now, ladies," said the lady sitting at the end of the desk. "How do you put the *fun* into funerals?"

The other ladies looked at each other like, *What?*

"Exactly! This is the bizarre story of Morag Walker, a single mum from outer London who has attended multiple funerals in recent months. The twist is – she wasn't invited to any of them!"

The audience gasped as one. That picture from *The Herald* appeared on the massive screen behind the presenters: Morag being held back, me attacking the security guards. That embarrassing pile of food next to Morag's empty handbag on the carpet.

"It seems that Ms Walker has been gatecrashing these funerals for the free food, the entertainment, and perhaps a bit of a pity party while she's at it. Her ruse was exposed last week when she crashed footballer Martin Winner's memorial service and security got wise."

"That is despicable," one of the other presenters said, shaking her head. "A funeral should be for friends and family to grieve, not for freeloaders to fill their pockets. In all my years on this show, I've honestly never heard of anything quite like it."

The picture of us disappeared from the screen and was replaced by shaky, close-up footage of Morag. I remembered it clearly. Morag looked smart; it was the day of the Bojangles interview. A microphone appeared in the shot, then Morag pushed it away. The camera wobbled, and Morag disappeared into Bojangles.

"And that's not all," the main presenter continued. "It appears that always in tow is her ten-year-old son, who is allegedly used as a distraction piece while Miss Walker stashes away free food and downs alcoholic drinks, on the house."

The five posh ladies tutted.

"Sad," one muttered. "Getting a child involved is really unfortunate."

"Does she need the food?" another asked. "Or is something else going on here?"

"She lost her job earlier this year," said the lady at the end. "Maybe this is a way to put food on the table. But does that make her behaviour ethical? Maureen, what's your take on this?"

"Surely there are services available to help people in these situations," replied the one called Maureen. "I think it's *despicable* that anyone would need to resort to turning up to wakes just for food…"

The sound of the telly faded to a ringing in my ears. My head started to throb.

"Not even that bad, you said?" Morag said. "That's not what they think."

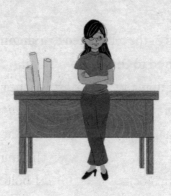

CHAPTER 19

Morag spent the night in her bedroom with the door closed.

She was still shut in there when I woke up the next morning. I knew she hadn't slept well. I could hear her rolling around in bed all night, the springs of her mattress groaning. I suppose I didn't sleep that well either.

Nothing felt real. I couldn't believe we'd been on the telly. I'd always wanted to be on the telly, but not like that. I never wanted to be on a show where they said mean things about Morag and showed a picture of me with a snail trail of snot dripping out of my nose.

All night I'd played it over and over in my head like

a video stuck on replay. The sound of the audience gasping in horror. *How do you put the fun into funerals?* The applause at the end of the advert break. *I've honestly never heard of anything quite like it.*

When I finally fell asleep, I dreamed about the gang of presenters with microphones chasing Morag and me round our block of flats, until I bolted upright in bed, shaking and covered in sweat.

I pushed my face into my pillow. At least no one was chucking eggs at the window. Yet.

"You're early, Solo!" Miss Carmichael said, shocked to see me just after the morning bell rang. "But we're still not *really* adhering to the school uniform policy, are we?"

Sometimes Miss Carmichael said "we" when she really meant "you". I think she thought it sounded nicer, when really she was just being mean.

I looked down at my clothes. I was so sleepy that I'd chucked on whatever I could grab without waking up Morag. Two odd socks, my funeral suit, my ropy school jumper and my old mud-caked trainers.

"That does mean another demerit as well as a letter home, I'm afraid, Solo. I know we can turn this round though. Don't forget to tell Mum about the uniform sale." She walked across the room and added another sticker to the chart. My snaking line of red demerit stickers reminded me of the dots the yellow character eats in that game *Pac-Man*. "The good news is that Mr Stephens has added a desk to Table C at the back."

I looked at Table C. A desk had been tacked on to the side at a weird angle so I was still basically sitting alone. Nobody on Table C looked happy that I was joining them.

Chetna turned and faced me once I'd sat down. "Are you OK? You really need to get your uniform sorted out, Solo."

"Cheers, *Star of the Week*," I grumbled. "I'm just waiting for Mor— I mean, my mum to get it for me."

"Well, tell her to hurry up because those trainers are *so* lame," Melissa butted in. "And odd socks? Really not today's vibe."

Chetna rolled her eyes, which made me feel better. Melissa was the worst. Actually, a lot of people in our class were the worst.

"Our collage looks super cool up there!" Chetna said, smiling at the wall.

She was right. It looked so vibrant. It was the best piece of work I had ever done. I wished I could take it home to show Morag, but she wouldn't care.

There was a knock on the classroom door. Miss Ellis appeared and beckoned Miss Carmichael over to the door, where they whispered secretively to each other. I couldn't help but notice that they kept glancing over at me. I pretended to concentrate on the floor.

"Solo Walker," Miss Carmichael called. "You're wanted in Mrs Howe's office – right now. Miss Ellis will walk you over."

Everyone went quiet and started gawping at me like I was a woolly mammoth back from the dead or something. Mrs Howe was the head teacher, and a summons to her office meant only one thing: I was in serious trouble. I could feel heat crawling up my neck.

"You've obviously made a *grave* mistake," Kai whispered, and all his cronies fell apart laughing.

"Kai Bailey," Miss Ellis called across the room. "I have reason to believe you smuggled a pair of craft scissors home yesterday after we completed the collages…"

Kai went oven-hob red. "No, Miss! What are you on about?"

"Oh, that's odd," said Miss Ellis. "Because your mum brought them into reception a minute ago.

She was quite apologetic, said it's becoming a bit of a habit. Just a reminder not to do it again please." She waved the scissors in her hand before passing them to Miss Carmichael.

A barely held-in smirk spread across the class. I had to force myself to keep a straight face because Kai looked like he was about to burst out crying.

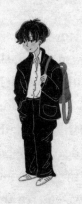

CHAPTER 20

Mrs Howe's office was silent and weird. It smelled like a mixture of coffee and the huge bunch of flowers that was sitting on her desk in a vase. They reminded me of the flowers at funerals, white and full of yellow powdery pollen.

I'd never been in Mrs Howe's office before, which surprised me as I wasn't well behaved. I guess I got away with stuff by sneaking under the radar like a submarine. You had to do something really bad to get noticed, like when Kai Bailey stole Aisha Gilmore's brand-new berry-scented crackle slime and got all the reception kids to eat it.

I hadn't done anything *that* bad, had I? I started to

worry. Maybe Mrs Howe knew about the pea-flicking incident. Or worse – maybe she knew about my trusty escape hole behind the canteen bins.

I swung my legs back and forth while I waited for Mrs Howe to appear. The chair in front of her desk was padded and made of soft fabric. It would have been comfortable if I hadn't been so nervous.

Finally Mrs Howe entered the room with a crash, almost dropping a box of folders all over the floor. She was still talking to her secretary, who was sitting outside the office. Mrs Howe didn't sound very happy.

"Well, tell them that maths is not an optional subject. If I don't see that boy back in class by next week, we will have to take further action with the local authorities."

I cleared my throat. It was too late to leg it now.

Just one second, she mouthed to me as she lingered by the door.

"Good," she said to her secretary. "Keep me posted. Bye."

Mrs Howe sighed and put down the box on her desk, then rubbed the sides of her head for a few seconds. It reminded me of Morag when she said she'd "had it up to here with my nonsense". Mrs Howe's hair was light brown with flecks of grey running through it. A bit like the red squirrels on our nature collage.

"Solo," she said, sitting down. "How are things?"

I swallowed. "Fine. Everything's fine."

"Everything all right at home?"

I nodded, probably too enthusiastically. "Everything's just great, Mrs Howe."

Mrs Howe paused as if she didn't know how to choose her next words. "I understand there's been a bit of fuss recently," she said. "Your mum has been in the news a bit."

"Oh, that." My mouth went as dry as the Sahara Desert and my face was as hot as the sun. "That was all a, erm, misunderstanding."

"Right." She stared into my eyes, as if searching for more answers. "Care to tell me what happened, Solo?"

"That funeral we were at, my mum *did* know the guy. Everyone's saying we weren't invited, but that's all wrong. It wasn't what it looked like!"

"I see." Mrs Howe looked suspicious. "Well, it sounds like a difficult situation, with the media being involved. You do know that if you or your mum ever need any support, we can help. I've tried your mum's mobile—"

"No!" I blurted out. "Everything's fine. Morag – I mean, Mum – was a bit too sad at the wake."

"Does that happen often, Solo?" She tilted her head. "Does Mum get a bit too sad a lot?"

"No!" I faked a laugh. "I told you. Everything. Is. Fine."

She chewed on her lip while she kept staring at me. "I want you to know where I am if there's ever anything we can do to help. Us teachers, we're not all evil, you know."

I smirked but kept it inside my head so Mrs Howe didn't notice. That's what *she* thought.

"I'll be making Miss Carmichael aware of the situation," Mrs Howe went on, "so she can keep an eye on things. Don't be afraid to ask her for anything you need, OK?"

"OK," I said, knowing I would never ask Miss Cowmichael for anything.

"She told me you're struggling with your uniform. We really do need to get this sorted, Solo. There's a reason we have a uniform policy. Believe it or not, it's for your own good. And that suit is … not school regulation. We do have grants and second-hand sales available to help with things like uniform, if your mum might be interested…"

"She knows," I said. "Mum is going to get the right uniform for me tomorrow from the shops, I promise. With the school logo and everything."

"OK, well, I do hope that's the case. I'll give you this to jog her memory, all right?" Mrs Howe slid a white envelope across the desk. It was addressed to *The Parents or Guardians of Solo Walker*. She gave me a tight smile. "Make sure she reads it."

"Yes, Mrs Howe."

I took the envelope, folded it and put it into my jacket pocket. I would decide later whether I was brave enough to show Morag.

"Keep your chin up, Solo," Miss Howe said as I left. "This too shall pass."

To be honest, I didn't have a clue what she was on about.

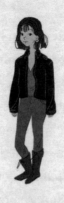

CHAPTER 21

"Oh, for Pete's sake." Morag screwed Mrs Howe's letter into a ball and launched it at the kitchen bin. She missed. "That's the last thing I need. Where am I supposed to get the money for this?"

"Sorry, Morag," I mumbled. I instantly regretted being brave and giving her the letter. "But you did say you'd get me a new uniform…"

"And I've told you I'm trying, haven't I?" She switched the kettle on, then flicked it off again. She was shaking and her skin was grey.

"Well, try harder!" I yelled.

I stormed into the bathroom and slammed the door. Our two toothbrushes rattled around in their cup on the sink.

I tried not to shout when Morag was feeling low, but sometimes I couldn't help it. The Reds could be contagious like chicken pox, and being so close to Morag meant that sometimes I caught the Reds from her.

I was the one getting called Funeral Boy. The whole thing was all her fault. If Morag hadn't got fired from her job at the train station, none of this would have happened.

"Solo." Morag rapped on the bathroom door. "I'm sorry. I'm just stressed right now, but it isn't your fault. Come on out, Solo."

"No. I don't want to talk to you, Morag!"

"Well, you can't stay in there for ever. What are you going to eat for dinner? Toothpaste? A bar of soap?"

I hated it when she did that. She always made me smile when I was trying my absolute best to stay angry.

She didn't stop there. "Moisturizer with a side of shower gel? Shampoo for dessert? Sounds pretty gross if you ask me."

I unlocked the door and let it swing open. Morag was sitting cross-legged on the floor. She looked guilty, which made me feel guilty too.

"Come here." She held her arms out, and I crawled into them slowly, pretending like I didn't want to.

"We'll get you your uniform, OK? Tomorrow."

"Really, Morag? Tomorrow?"

"Really," she said. "I promise."

I looked at Morag right in the eyes. "But how will you get the money?"

"You know me," she said. "I'll figure something out."

"Are you sure?"

"Surely sure I'm sure," she said.

It was a thing we did. Only this time, Morag didn't look sure at all.

The uniform shop was called Meagre and Jones School Attire Emporium, and it stank of dust and old cupboards. They also sold toys, games and books, but Morag said I wasn't allowed to look at that stuff because she didn't want any pestering from the likes of me.

It was weird looking at all the other school uniforms that were available. They had rails and rails of jumpers and blazers, hanging all the way up to the ceiling. Each uniform was like a different life I could've had, with no Miss Cowmichael, no Kai Bailey, and no Melissa Underwood always accusing me of fancying her.

I wondered what other schools were like. Did they

have lockers in the halls like in America? Were there swimming pools and AstroTurf football pitches? I'd heard some schools went abroad on school trips, like to Africa to see the safari animals. I guessed I would never do anything like that.

But I had to admit school wasn't *all* bad. Things had improved since Chetna had arrived. And Miss Ellis had stuck up for me twice now. Plus, I couldn't wait to see Miss Cowmichael's face when I came in wearing my smart new uniform, complete with the official logo.

The only thing missing was the shoes, but we would sort those out another time, Morag said. Shoes were expensive.

Normally I hated trying on clothes, but this time I relished it. Morag kept asking how it was looking through the curtain, but I couldn't reply. I just kept staring into the mirror.

This jumper had no holes, and the trousers ended at my ankles rather than hanging over my shoes. I ran my fingers over the stitched school logo on the blazer, feeling the thickness of the embroidery. It felt new and pristine, not a stain or mark to be seen.

"Look at my handsome grown-up boy!" Morag squealed when I pulled back the curtain. It was embarrassing but I didn't tell her off. She made me twirl round, which made me go red because I wasn't a ballerina.

"Just enough growing room there," said the shopkeeper, who looked oddly like Santa. "Should see him through to the end of Year Six, no trouble."

"Brilliant," Morag said. "What's the damage then, for the full set?"

"With the two shirts, that'll be one hundred and seventeen pounds, twelve pence."

Morag went greyer than usual and cleared her throat. "How about with just the one shirt?"

I went back into the changing room and put my normal clothes back on, taking care to fold my new uniform properly on the stool. When I came back out, Morag was flicking through the cards in her wallet.

"Why don't you go and wait outside for Mummy, sweetheart? I won't be a minute."

I rolled my eyes. She was doing the old "Mummy" trick again.

Outside, I scuffed my shoes to pass the time and watched pigeons pecking at crumbs on the ground. Morag was taking ages, and I was starting to need a wee. I was about to go back in and ask what was taking so long when I heard shouting.

"Hey!" I heard the shopkeeper yell. "What do you think you're doing?"

Morag burst through the doors with the new uniform bundled under her arm like a rugby ball.

I turned to her. "What's—"

"I'll explain later," she panted, grabbing my wrist and dragging me along behind her. "Just run, Solo! Run!"

I looked back. The shopkeeper was out on the street, shaking his fists, and he seemed red in the face. He chased us for a bit, then gave up.

"I know who you are, you funeral-crashers! You'll pay for this!"

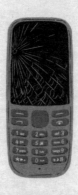

CHAPTER 22

Morag rummaged through the kitchen drawers looking for her little black notebook while I caught my breath at the table. I had never run so fast in my life. All the way from the shops and back home, never stopping to walk, never looking behind us. My lungs were burning and my legs felt numb.

"*Meagre and Jones School Attire Emporium...*" Morag mumbled as she wrote, breathing heavily. "*One hundred and seventeen pounds, twelve pence...*"

It was the latest in a list of restaurants and shops and supermarkets that she'd borrowed from, usually without asking permission first. Noodle Town restaurant, the corner shop, the chemist down the road. The list went back for pages and pages, starting when she first lost her job.

"When I'm rich," she said as she returned the small notebook to the drawer, "I'll make sure everyone gets every single penny and more."

"Yeah, I know," I said, turning on the telly. Morag had been saying the same thing for ages. I had no idea if she really meant it, or when she planned to be rich. I only wished she would hurry up with that particular plan.

My new uniform was strewn over the arm of the sofa, but it didn't feel the same as it did when I tried it on in the shop. Somehow it felt dirtier than my ragged old funeral suit. It felt grubby without there being a single stain.

"I worked up quite a sweat there," Morag puffed. "I haven't had a workout that good in a long time. I'll go have a shower. Just … don't watch the news, OK?"

I nodded. I switched to a cartoon about some animal detectives that I was too old for while Morag turned on the shower. The pipes screeched and groaned as the water rushed through. She started singing to herself as she got clean.

Morag's phone buzzed on the kitchen table. Then again. And again. I tiptoed into the dark kitchen and peered at the cracked screen.

Is this you? a message read. It was sent by someone called Mark Work, probably someone from her old job. It was followed by a link. Is everything OK?

Then another from somebody else: Everyone's talking about you... You're a hashtag!

Shaking, I unlocked Morag's phone and clicked the link in the first message. It led to a site full of different names and faces. I scrolled down, then down again. Everyone was reposting that picture of Morag and me from the wake. Sick started bubbling in my stomach.

Elizabeth @MrsTwinkle1974 14:18
Wow. Just wow. The things people will do for a free meal! #FuneralMum #FuneralBoy

Jim @JimTheSparky7 14:07
Why is nobody talking about Martin Winner the #LuckyStriker? #FuneralMum has really stolen the limelight from this titan of football.

Tuna @TunaMeltConnoisseur 14:04
Does anyone know anything about #FuneralBoy? Is he OK living with #FuneralMum?

Dave @LactoseIntolerantLad 13:57
Will be keeping an eye out for #FuneralMum
and #FuneralBoy at the mother-in-law's memorial
service tomorrow. #StayVigilant #FuneralCrashing
#Scam

Mariella @MistleToe43 13:49
This might be bad but I can't stop creasing at
#FuneralBoy's face. That snot bubble – Gross!

Tom @TwistedLibrarian89 13:34
I stand in support of #FuneralMum. Why not
make funerals a bit more fun? Load of fuss over
nothing if you ask me.

Mickey @MickeyUnderwood78 13:29
#FuneralBoy goes to school with my daughter.
Bit weird apparently, spends half the time hiding
in the cloakroom! Daughter has tried to be
friends but no luck #BeKind

Kingsley @KingsleyT 13:22
I might be wrong but I'm pretty sure
#FuneralMum is my neighbour! Hope they're OK
#FuneralBoy

Colin @Meagre&JonesSchoolwear 13:10

#FuneralMum and #FuneralBoy were just in the store and made off without paying! Law enforcement *will* be involved!

I scrolled and scrolled but the page went on for ever. When I thought I'd reached the bottom, more loaded. More pictures, more words, more anonymous profiles gossiping about me and Morag.

"What are you doing with my phone?" Morag was behind me in her polka-dot dressing gown, water dripping from her hair and on to the floor.

I dropped the phone on the kitchen table like a hot piece of coal. "Nothing! I—"

Morag grabbed the phone and started scrolling, the light of the screen illuminating her wide eyes.

"You're joking me," she muttered, then she started to tremble. "You have got to be kidding me."

"Don't read it, Morag!" I swiped the phone from her hand. "They don't know us. You always tell me not to listen to people who don't know me!"

"Give me that!" she snarled, snatching it back again.

"Just don't, Morag!" I tried to wrestle it free of her hand, but her grip was iron tight.

Then, in the blink of an eye, Morag raised the

phone high above her head and launched it against the kitchen wall. The phone bounced and skidded across the floor. A huge crack spread across the screen.

Everything went quiet. Everything was still.

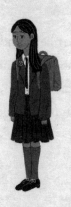

CHAPTER 23

"Well, who's this dapper young man at the door?" Miss Carmichael cooed as I arrived in class the next morning. "That's one green mark for nearly perfect uniform! I'll even forgive the trainers on this occasion."

I went bright red, obviously. My new shirt collar was too stiff, and my trousers were itchy and rough against my legs.

"*Pfft.* Still a weirdo though, aren't you? New uniform or not," Kai Bailey whispered as I went to my desk. "Hashtag Funeral Boy."

Chetna turned to face me, beaming. "Looking super sharp, Solo!" She gave me two thumbs up. "You'll be up for Star of the Week if you keep this up!"

Our task that morning was to make a smoothie that was both delicious *and* nutritious from the ingredients on the whiteboard at the front of the class. Miss Carmichael kept repeating "delicious *and* nutritious" as if it was some sort of funny joke, but it was only a rhyme, and nobody laughed.

Chetna and I were in a pair again. We decided to make a smoothie called a Monkey Flip, which Chetna said she'd had in a cafe with her parents one time. It had milk, banana, peanut butter, dates and then a huge dollop of syrup to actually make it delicious.

When Chetna went to the toilet, I secretly added two more spoonfuls of syrup to the mixture. I thought it would make it taste even better, but Chetna said it kind of ruined the smoothie because it was too sweet. I said too sweet isn't possible, which Chetna found funny. The drink was still nice enough, and we slurped our smoothies right up.

Miss Carmichael said our smoothie could have been a tiny bit more nutritious, but it was definitely delicious, which was good enough for me. First the collage, then the uniform, now this. I was starting to worry that I was enjoying school.

I was sucking the last dregs through my reusable

straw when Miss Ellis appeared at the door and glanced my way. Again? My winning streak hadn't lasted long at all.

"Solo Walker?" she said into the room. She beckoned to me. "Come with me to Mrs Howe's office, if you don't mind. Bring your bag."

"What have you done this time?" Chetna asked. "So much for Star of the Week."

"I have no idea!" I whispered, gathering up my things.

Miss Ellis's sandals made a slapping sound as we walked the corridors to Mrs Howe's office.

"How's things?" she said after a while. "Have those girls given you any more bother?"

"Not really," I said. "But they don't exactly like me either."

"Well, do you want them to like you?" she said. "Because maybe you just have to learn to tolerate each other. Not everybody's meant to be best buddies."

I nodded. I'd never thought about it like that, but it sounded pretty smart. Plus, I had Chetna now, so I didn't even care about the Cool Table.

"Did you pass on that information about the food bank to Mum?"

"Yeah…" I swallowed. My throat was dry.

"And?"

"She said she'd think about it." I didn't have the heart to tell Miss Ellis that the leaflet and voucher she had given me were currently crumpled in a ball at the bottom of our kitchen bin.

"Great! I also wanted to give you this." Miss Ellis dug through her shoulder bag and produced a bulky carrier bag. She looked kind of embarrassed as she gave it to me. "Don't worry if you don't like them. I won't be offended."

"What is it?" I said, confused. I hadn't asked anyone for anything, and it definitely wasn't my birthday.

"Just open it – you'll see."

I stopped and looked inside it, to find a cardboard box. Inside that were sheets of brown packing paper and then a pair of smart black shoes.

"What?" I spluttered. "Why?"

"School shoes," she said, blushing a bit. "I know you've been getting a hard time about the trainers. I guessed you were a size four…"

My mouth hung open. I didn't know what to say.

"You don't have to take them home if you don't want to. You can leave them in my cupboard and put them on in the morning if you like. It's always unlocked."

I turned the shoes over in my hands, inspecting them. They were black with Velcro straps and stitched stripes running down the outer sides. They smelled like brand-new leather and shoe polish. They were so shiny I could actually see my reflection in them.

"Who paid for these?" I said.

"Well…" Miss Ellis sort of coughed a bit. "I did. But it doesn't matter. It's a gift. To get people off your back a bit. Go on – put them on … if you like."

I took off my trainers and squeezed my feet into the new shoes without even undoing the straps. They fitted perfectly and looked so smart.

"Thanks, Miss Ellis," I said. "They're brilliant. Are you *sure*?"

Miss Ellis smiled. "Very sure. Now come on – Mrs Howe will be waiting."

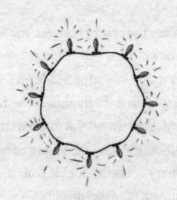

CHAPTER 24

"Ah, here you are, young Mr Walker," Mrs Howe said. "Smart uniform, by the way."

"Thanks, Miss. I mean, Missus… I mean, Mrs Howe."

She smiled at me, but somehow didn't seem very happy.

"Did Mum take you shopping? Meagre and Jones, by any chance?"

I froze like a dummy in a shop window. My ears started to throb.

"Why don't you take a seat, Solo?" Mrs Howe spun round her computer screen so I could see it, and clicked to enlarge a video. "There's something I want to show you."

Immediately I put my head in my hands and

watched through the cracks between my fingers. This was going to be painful.

There was me in a grainy black-and-white video recording, filmed from high above. Me handing my uniform to Morag while she flicked through her wallet. Then Morag telling me to go and wait outside. Then me, blurry, outside, kicking at the floor and messing about with the pigeons.

"Stop," I said. "I don't want to—"

But the video continued. There was Morag, looking over her shoulder before pointing to something behind the counter. There was the shopkeeper turning away to fetch it, then Morag sprinting out of the door, dragging me away with her.

Mrs Howe turned the screen back to face her, then let out a long and disappointed sigh.

I didn't speak. I didn't move. There was nothing I could say.

"I've had Colin Meagre, the shop owner, on the phone today. It's fair to say he's rather upset with you and your mum, Solo. It's really not acceptable what's happened here."

I didn't know what to say. I suddenly felt too hot. I felt trapped. I wanted to escape but I felt superglued to the seat.

"I regret that I'm having to bring this up with you, Solo," said Mrs Howe gently. "We would have much rather discussed this with your mum, but she hasn't been answering the phone."

I looked at my hands, then the window, then the plant in the corner. Anything to avoid Mrs Howe's gaze.

"The owners chose to contact us rather than going to the police," she said quietly.

The police. I swallowed and blinked at the floor. "Are we going to prison?"

Mrs Howe sort of laughed, but not really. "No, no. Mr Meagre seems very reasonable, all things considered. If your mum can bring in the money as soon as possible, he's willing to keep this quiet."

I let out all the air I'd been holding in my body. I was worried I was about to get arrested and dragged away by a team of police officers in front of the whole school.

"Typically we would consider speaking to social services at this point," Mrs Howe continued, "but I don't want to make things worse, not with everything else going on." She tapped on her keyboard, then showed me Morag's number on the computer screen. "Is this the right number for her?"

"Yeah." I gritted my teeth. "Sorry, Mrs Howe. I'll tell her you called."

"And, Solo…" she said. "If money is an issue, we can help. The uniform need not cost an arm and a leg. There are ways we can support families with things like this. All we'd need to do is speak to your mum—"

"I said I'll tell her!" I blurted out. I just wanted to get out of there. "I'll get it sorted."

"Understood." Mrs Howe looked at her computer screen. "Well, you know where I am, Solo."

Outside, I crawled through my secret escape hole in the fence behind the canteen bins and ran. Morag had to know about the shopkeeper right now, or our lives were about to get a hundred times worse. People dodged me as I sprinted home, my backpack flailing from shoulder to shoulder. I swore I heard somebody shout, "Isn't that Funeral Boy?" But I didn't have time to care, not any more.

The flat was all dark and quiet. No lights on. No cooking sounds or smells coming from the kitchen. No laughter or talking blaring from the telly. No Morag singing to herself in the shower. Not even her slow, huffing snores like when she was asleep.

"Morag? Are you here?"

I went into her bedroom, where I thought she could be hiding under the duvet. When I ripped it off Morag's bed, a mountain of laundry was underneath. The room was a total tip, with loads of cups and bottles everywhere. Morag's clothes were scattered all over the floor. The air smelled funny, like the window hadn't been opened in a year. Her room was always a bit like this when she had the Big Bad Reds. But it wasn't normally this bad.

Next, I went into the bathroom, ripping back the shower curtain, but nothing nor no one greeted me other than the slow *drip, drip, drip* of the leaky shower and our two toothbrushes standing side by side in their cup.

She wasn't in the living room either, and she definitely wasn't in the kitchen, even though I looked in all the cupboards and under the table, as if we were playing a silly game of hide-and-seek.

"Morag?" I croaked. "Morag?"

I tried my best to calm down. Maybe she had gone to the shop for more of her grown-up drinks. Or maybe she'd gone out for a walk and forgotten the time.

Horrible thoughts that usually stayed in the back of my mind kept barging to the front. What if Morag didn't come back? What if Morag had decided she didn't like me any more and run away? What if the police had already come for Morag and taken her away?

It was all my fault. All my fault for nagging her about my uniform, even though I knew she didn't have the money.

Suddenly a buzzing sound shattered the silence. Chills skittered down my spine like spiders. Morag's phone. I ran into the bedroom, where the phone was juddering on the bedside table.

"Hello?" I said, swiping my finger across the cracked screen. My heart sank in my chest; I hated talking on the phone. "Morag? Is that you?"

"Hello, I'm looking to speak with Morag Walker?" The voice at the end of the phone sounded very posh and smarmy. "My name's Jack Morley. I'm calling from the *Daily News* head office in London."

"Oh," I said. My mind was racing. *The* Daily News? *Head office?* It all sounded too serious. "Morag isn't here right now, sorry," I replied, trembling. "She… She's gone to the shops!"

"No bother. It's about this funeral business. We wanted to get in touch to hear her side of the story. Perhaps a tell-all interview could be on the cards?"

"S-sorry," I said. "I've got to go now. Bye."

"Is this Solo Walker speaking? The boy from the photo? We could even chat to you too. This could be a fantastic opportunity to set the record straight."

The phone beeped as I pressed the "end call" button. I didn't like the sound of that man at all. Morag always said that you shouldn't trust posh people.

I tucked the phone into my pocket and walked back into the kitchen to get a glass of squash.

And then I saw something that made me stop dead in my tracks.

I hadn't noticed it all the time I'd been searching. I'd been in too much of a panic. Right there in the middle of the messy kitchen table was a note in Morag's scribbly handwriting. It only had six words.

I can't do this any more.

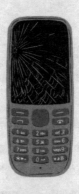

CHAPTER 25

I can't do this any more.

I threw Morag's phone on to the sofa and paced around the living room. It was eight o'clock at night. It was so quiet I could hear my pulse hammering.

It wasn't the first time that the Big Bad Reds had caused Morag to go missing. When Dad first went away, Morag left me all alone in the flat for almost a whole day.

It wasn't as bad as it sounds. There was plenty of food in the cupboards back then, and enough cartoons on the telly to make the time go quickly. I actually had a really good time with no Morag bossing me about. It was like being a grown-up – pure freedom.

The worst bit was tucking myself into bed. I

preferred it when Morag stuck her head over the top of the sofa and reminded me why I was called Solo. Come to think of it, Morag hadn't done that in a while.

Anyway, that first time, Morag came back eventually, acting cheery as anything. She had a new haircut and a load of new clothes she couldn't afford. Said she'd needed a bit of retail therapy. It was like nothing had ever happened in the first place.

She took me to Noodle Town for a meal to say sorry, and we had a special party, just the two of us. When we got back to the flat we had the radio on and danced. Morag spun me around like we were in a movie.

She made me promise never to tell a soul that she had left me on my own. Apparently, if anyone found out, they'd put me in a home, and neither of us wanted that.

It's our secret, Morag would say, tapping the side of her nose. *Mum's the word, Solo. Mum's the word.*

Which meant I shouldn't tell anyone she was gone now.

I took Morag's crumpled note out of my pocket and read it one more time. *I can't do this any more.* I folded the note back into a neat square and put it back in my pocket with the phone. More little secrets for me to carry around.

*

Dinner was made of whatever bits I could chuck together from the kitchen. I had a crumpet with butter, a packet of salt-and-vinegar crisps, some dry frosted cornflakes. Dessert was a slightly fizzy yoghurt that had been in the fridge too long. As Miss Carmichael would say, it was neither delicious nor nutritious.

Even though I missed Morag, it was kind of fun making dinner. I walked around the kitchen like I owned the place, even wiping up my crumbs with a cloth and sprinkling them into the bin. I forgot about Morag for a few minutes while I concentrated on putting the food in a nice circle on the plate.

I ate it with whatever cutlery I liked. Morag's favourite knife with the leopard-print design. My favourite fork with the dinosaur-head handle. They were completely mismatched, just like Morag and Dad. I put my plate in the sink when I was done, but I didn't wash it up because that was Morag's job.

I put the telly on extra loud to take my mind off things. There were all sorts of grown-up shows on that I wasn't allowed to watch. Shows about the police catching criminals and people swearing. It was fun for a bit, but I kept getting nervous that Morag would come home and catch me red-handed.

At around two o'clock in the morning, my eyes felt heavy. I made sure the front door was unlocked for Morag and pulled the curtains across the eggy windows.

With Morag's phone still heavy as a stone in my pocket, I crawled under my duvet and pulled it close to stay warm all night long. I listened to the sounds of cars and buses rushing past the flat, crashing over speed bumps. I wondered where they were all going at this time so late, or so early.

I closed my eyes and tried to let the sound lull me into a shallow sleep.

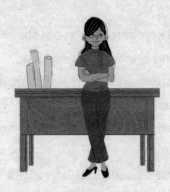

CHAPTER 26

Worst sleep ever. If I could even call it sleep.

All night long I had nightmares about Morag. About Morag never coming back home and me having to live on my own for ever. About Morag getting caught by the police for some terrible crime and going to jail for the rest of her life. I dreamed about a fancy funeral, where everyone stared at Morag and me and counted every bit of food we ate. I dreamed about a camera flashing bright white in my eyes, blinding me.

I jolted awake. Morag's phone was vibrating in my pyjama pocket.

"Morag?" I gasped. "Are you there?"

"Good morning, Solo!" The voice sounded upbeat.

"Jack Morley from the *Daily News* again. Any thoughts on that interview?"

"Leave us alone!" I shouted. "Morag doesn't want to do your stupid interview, got it?"

Jack sighed. "Look, just put her on the line for me, OK? This is grown-up chat. They do say never work with kids and animals—"

"Morag's not here!" I blurted out, before clapping a hand over my mouth in shock.

"Well, where is she? I'd prefer to speak to her today—"

"I don't know where she is!" I snapped. Again, immediately I regretted it. "I haven't seen her since yesterday. There – happy now?" *Why couldn't I stop talking?!*

There was silence on the other end of the call. My thoughtless words lingered between us.

"Do you mean to tell me your mum's gone missing?" the journalist asked slowly.

I hung up the call.

I put on my stolen uniform. I was so tired that my arms and legs felt heavier than usual. I felt like I was wading through treacle. Normally it took ten minutes to walk to school, but today it took twenty, even in the new shoes Miss Ellis had given me.

"Keeping you up, are we?" Miss Carmichael joked, as I walked into class yawning. I hated it when teachers said that. I always wanted to say, *Yes, you are keeping me up, actually. I'd much rather be in my nice warm bed, dreaming good dreams, and not at school.*

Everything Miss Carmichael said in English class just turned into muffled nonsense in my ears. The writing on the board seemed to scramble and scuttle around like insects.

"Any thoughts, Mr Sleepyhead at the back?"

Everyone looked at me. I clamped my mouth shut, stifling down another yawn. "Sorry, Miss."

"You're absolutely yawning your head off, Solo! I know sentence structures aren't the most thrilling of subjects, but try to stay with us."

"Sorry, Miss," I said again. "I didn't sleep very well last night."

Everyone giggled. No matter what I said, everyone giggled. *Maybe I should become a comedian*, I thought. Everything I did was *just so funny*.

"What time did you go to bed?" Miss Carmichael asked.

"About midnight." I went red and stared at the

floor. I wasn't going to tell her that it was more like two o'clock in the morning.

"That's not enough sleep for a boy your age," she said. "I'll chat to your mum about it."

"She'll probably be too drunk to care," Kai Bailey hissed from across the class.

"Shut up, Kai," I snapped, without really meaning to. "At least my mum doesn't look like a giant *rat* like yours. Must be where you get it from."

Everyone made a noise like, *Ooooooh!*

"BOYS, THAT'S ENOUGH." Miss Carmichael was doing the face where her jaw stuck out and her nostrils flared as wide as Underground train tunnels.

I sighed, ready to get my head bitten off by Miss Carmichael.

"Kai Bailey, I've had just about enough of your sly, immature comments," Miss Carmichael snapped, clapping her hands loudly. "Learn when to zip your mouth up, or you'll find yourself languishing outside Mrs Howe's office for the rest of the week."

Kai's eyes went all red. It was brilliant. I couldn't believe she wasn't shouting at *me*. But then she turned round.

"The same goes for you, Solo Walker. Keep it in the playground, or better – nowhere at all."

"But he started it!" I protested.

"Two wrongs don't make a right, not in my classroom. That's a demerit for the pair of you for being disruptive during lesson time."

I put my head down again and stared at the table. Miss Carmichael carried on with the lesson, writing on the board way more aggressively than normal. The pen was actually squeaking so much it was like it was telling us off itself.

"Whatever's going on with you, you need to snap out of it, Solo." Chetna sat beside me on the cloakroom bench while everyone else played outside. "Otherwise Miss Carmichael will never give you a break."

Part of me wanted to be on my own, to sort everything out in my head. But the other part was desperate for somebody to talk to. Somebody to ask what on earth I should do.

"She just hates me, that's what it is. Always has, always will."

"She doesn't *hate* you," she said. "She wants you to follow the rules. She is a *teacher*, after all."

Chetna's voice sounded kind of posh sometimes, like she was already a grown-up. I wasn't sure whether Morag would like her or not. Chetna didn't sound anything like we did. She sounded clever.

"She's a total cow," I said. "That's why everyone calls her Miss *Cow*michael." I slumped back against the coats and bags that hung behind me.

Chetna giggled, but checked around to make sure nobody had caught her doing it. "That is a pretty funny nickname, I suppose. What's up today? You seem … weird."

"How would you know? I only met you this week."

Chetna went a bit red then, and I felt bad. "No need to be horrible, Solo. I was just saying."

I looked at Chetna. Morag would kill me if I told anyone she was gone. But something about Chetna's friendly brown eyes made me feel like I could trust her.

I sighed. "I'm just worried about something, that's all."

"Oh, go on, you have to tell me! I'm great at solving problems. I've got my problem-solving certificate and everything. They say a problem shared is a problem halved, you know."

I didn't know if that was true. Whenever I shared a problem, it seemed to grow to twice the size. Like years ago, when I told Morag about the Year Four boy who kept flicking me on the forehead whenever we played outside at break. At pick-up time she found the boy's mum and flicked her so hard on the forehead that they had a massive argument in the playground. Next thing I knew, Mrs Howe got involved and everyone found out that I'd snitched. Since then, I had tried to keep things to myself.

"I can't tell you, Chetna. I can't tell *anyone* – that's the thing."

"I promise I won't tell. Pinky swear?"

We linked our pinkies again and rattled the chain.

"Is it the whole hashtag Funeral Boy thing? Because that isn't your fault. I personally don't ever call you Funeral Boy. I think it's a *stupid* nickname, even if everyone else on the Cool Table—"

I shook my head. I didn't know where to start.

"You can tell me, Solo. Everybody says I'm a great pair of ears." Chetna pushed her ears forward so she looked goofy.

I laughed. "So you still haven't caved in to the scented-gel-pen craze?"

She shrugged. "Well, maybe one or two. I couldn't resist the blueberry. But I only use it ironically."

"What does *ironically* mean?"

Chetna wafted my question away with her hand. "Stop stalling. Now tell me what's going on."

I took Morag's mobile phone and the crinkled note

out of my pocket. There was still nothing from Morag. Missed calls flashed up on the screen: two seemed to be from the *Daily News*, and loads more from a contact called "Solo's School". Mrs Howe had been calling about the uniform.

"What's that?" Chetna asked, eyes widening. "You've got a *phone*? We're not allowed phones in school – it says so in the school handbook!"

"It's not mine. It's my mum's," I said, turning it over and over in my hand.

I took a deep breath.

"She's … missing." I swallowed. "I don't know where she is." I stuffed the note and phone back into my pocket. "But I'm sure it's fine. She's done it before and she came back."

Chetna looked scared. "You need to tell Miss Carmichael, Solo. What if something *happens*?" When I didn't answer, she said, "I'm sorry, but I might have to tell her myself."

"But you promised, remember? We pinky swore and everything!"

"Fine. But if she isn't back by tomorrow, we're telling Miss Carmichael. This is a big deal, Solo. Even if you try to pretend it isn't. Why have you got your mum's phone, anyway?"

"In case Morag calls her own number looking for me. Plus, there's games on there too."

Chetna smiled. "Don't tell anyone, but I have one too. Mum and Dad got it for me, but I'm only supposed to use it in emergencies." She rummaged in her bag and produced a pink smartphone with a glittery charm dangling from the corner. "Unlike *you*, I keep mine switched off and in my bag during school hours to avoid distractions." She shoved the phone back into her bag and checked around again.

"So you're not such a Little Miss Perfect after all?" I stuck my tongue out, and we both burst out laughing.

"Seriously, Solo," she said afterwards. "If your mum isn't back by tomorrow, we need to tell."

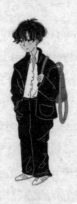

CHAPTER 27

"Solo," Miss Carmichael said, as soon as I walked back into class after lunch. "Can I have a quick word outside?"

A chill ran from my head to my toes. She knew about Morag's phone, I could tell. But how? I tucked the phone into my waistband, and hid that beneath my blazer.

"Everyone else, heads down," she said to the class. "You can work on finishing your acrostic poems from yesterday. I don't want to hear a peep from any of you while I'm gone!"

"*Yes, Miss Carmichael*," everybody droned.

Miss Carmichael walked out of the classroom without talking, and I followed behind. Her trainers squeaked on the corridor floors, and her bracelets jangled with the movement of her arms.

"You're not in any trouble," she eventually said, breaking the silence. "Let's go and find a quiet spot in the library and have a little chat, just you and me." I didn't believe her. I'd fallen for that one before. *You're not in trouble* usually meant *You're in massive trouble but we don't want you to leg it.*

In the library, Miss Carmichael found two chairs in a corner of the non-fiction section, next to the books about the Aztecs.

"Take a seat, Solo," she said, gesturing at one of the empty chairs. "Make yourself at home."

I sat down and trained my vision at the wooden table between us. No eye contact meant no mind-reading. I didn't really think Miss Carmichael could read minds, but I couldn't be too careful.

I decided to get in first. "Is this about earlier with Kai? Because if it is, he started it. He's always starting things with me."

Miss Carmichael nodded. "I know he started it, Solo. Trust me, I'll be having a separate conversation with Kai about his behaviour. But, no, that's not what this is about. I wanted to have a chat about how things are at home."

My mind went totally blank, like a new page in a notebook.

"Fine," I said. "Everything's absolutely fine."

"You don't have to put on a brave face, Solo. You can be honest with me."

"I am being honest, Miss," I said, blushing.

"I've been chatting with Miss Ellis and Mrs Howe. We know you've been in the news. Would you like to tell me anything about that?"

"That was a misunderstanding!" I said, pretending to be outraged. "My mum knew the guy whose funeral it was. They were mates."

"The article in *The Herald* seemed to imply that it was some sort of regular occurrence, and that they weren't mates, Solo. The article made it sound like your mum goes to an awful lot of funerals…"

"It's not." I shook my head. "And she doesn't."

"OK." Miss Carmichael nodded slowly. She kept twiddling with her bracelets. "We've tried to call your mum to discuss things, but I'm having a hard time getting an answer. There are resources we can direct you to. Food banks—"

"She's not interested," I blurted out. "She says we don't need it. Says she can cope fine."

Miss Carmichael nodded again. "It must be

difficult for you, being in the papers. There's an awful lot of unkindness out there."

"Most of it coming from Kai Bailey," I grumbled. "And everyone on the Cool Table. Except Chetna. Chetna's really nice."

"I'm glad you're getting along with Chetna. I've noticed the two of you talking. Don't worry about the rest of them, Solo. I see everything that happens in my classroom. It's like I've got eyes in the back of my head!"

A silence passed between us where Miss Carmichael probably expected me to laugh.

"And how is your mum, Solo?" asked Miss Carmichael. "I don't think I've seen or heard from her in quite some time."

"She's OK," I lied. "She's been busy, trying to find another job since she got fired from the train station."

"It's tough out there right now," Miss Carmichael said. "I think everyone's feeling the pinch. And how is she doing … otherwise?"

I screwed up my face involuntarily. "What do you mean, *otherwise*?"

Miss Carmichael was the one blushing now. "You know, generally."

"Morag's fine," I said. Morag wouldn't want me to tell Miss Carmichael the truth. "She just wants everything to blow over. She just wants everything to go back to normal."

Miss Carmichael nodded. "That it will, Solo. Just so you know, we're here to help if either of you need anything. Don't be scared to speak up."

"I won't, Miss," I said.

But there was no way I was doing that any time soon.

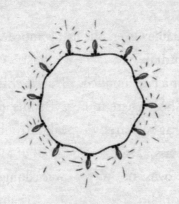

CHAPTER 28

At the sound of the bell, I sprinted away from school, desperate to know whether Morag had reappeared. I must have got home in record time.

Crossing my fingers, I bounded upstairs to our flat. I pictured Morag standing there in the kitchen, bundling me into the biggest hug ever.

I opened the front door. Cold. Dark. Silence. The only sound I could hear was Mr Thurston's TV playing from across the hallway.

"Morag? Are you there?" I called out hopefully. But I already knew the answer perfectly well. She wasn't.

The flat was exactly the same as when I'd left for school that morning. The curtains were still drawn; everything was dark. My bed was scruffy and unmade.

The kitchen table was covered in escaped bits of cereal from where I'd made myself breakfast.

There was a twisting feeling in my chest. I think it was worry. The longer she was away, the more likely it was that Morag was in some kind of trouble.

I kept seeing pictures in my head of Morag on the pavement in town begging for spare change. Or maybe she was in a pub with some new "friends" who she didn't even know properly.

Worse than that, what if she had met some new man and was busy being his new girlfriend and having a new baby and forgetting all about stupid Solo?

I got out Morag's phone. The sharp glass scratched my thumb as I swiped to activate the screen. Nothing from her. Only more missed calls from school and Jack Morley, and a warning that the battery was low.

In Morag's bedroom I found the charger and plugged in her phone. I stared hard at it, begging it to start ringing. The screen went black. I saw my shattered reflection in the glass.

I flattened out Morag's note again, to check for the hundredth time whether I had missed anything: a secret meaning to the words, or clues on the back of the paper that I hadn't noticed. It was starting to go soft between my fingers.

I can't do this any more. The words hadn't changed. There were no clues.

I crawled into Morag's bed, still wearing my uniform and pushed my face into the pillow. It smelled like Morag's strawberry shampoo. If I closed my eyes and imagined my hardest, she was there, calling me her special boy, reminding me why she chose to name me Solo.

Come on, Morag, I thought. *You have to come home.* I repeated the thought until my bones felt heavy, as though they were made of stone. Sleep came without me noticing and stayed for the weekend like an annoying guest in the flat. Without Morag, there was nothing to do but doze and watch the telly. I didn't dare go outside in case Morag arrived home and I wasn't there to hug her. The weekend had never felt so long.

On Sunday evening, a gentle knock at the door woke me up.

I heaved myself out of Morag's bed. I peered through the spyhole, and my heart sank down to the seams of my socks.

It was posh Mr Thurston from across the hall.

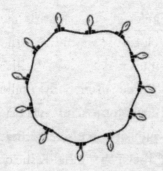

CHAPTER 29

"Evening, neighbour."

I had opened the door a crack. Mr Thurston was wearing a smart navy suit that fitted better than my funeral suit. He had curly hair with gel in it and wore aftershave that I could almost smell through the door.

"Listen, err," he said, "it's probably none of my business, but I just wanted to check on you and your mum. I'd seen you'd been getting a bit of –" he swallowed – "*unkindness* on the internet. To say the least."

"Oh," I replied, surprised. I thought he was here to tell me off about the ever-growing pile of unopened letters addressed to Morag by the main front door.

"We're fine, thanks."

"I'm Kingsley, by the way. I live across the hall. In flat nine."

"*Kingsley*," I said to nobody in particular. I'd assumed Mr Thurston's name would be Kenneth or Kevin or Keith or some sensible name that men in suits had. I'd seen the initial K in the post pile in the hall. I opened the door a bit wider. "I've seen you through the spyhole."

He laughed. "Ah, been watching me, have you?"

"No, no!" I said, going red.

He held both his palms up towards me. "I'm only messing. Anyway, is there anything you need?"

"Like what?"

"Oh, I don't know. Food … I could do a bit of shopping for you both?" He looked past me into the hall. "Is your mum around now?"

"No!" I pushed the door shut slightly, to stop him seeing into the flat. "She's out at the moment. She'll be back in a bit. I can tell her you came over."

Just then, my stomach let out the most embarrassing noise. It sounded like a cross between the last bit of a bath running down the plug and a whale singing under the ocean.

Mr Thurston – Kingsley – looked at me, wide-eyed.

"Wow. That was quite the stomach rumble. Have you eaten?"

I nodded, but my stomach betrayed me and gurgled again at the mere mention of food.

"Sounds like you're Hank Marvin to me," he said.

"My name's actually Solo Walker," I said, confused. "Not Hank Marvin."

"I know." He smiled. "Ignore me. Why don't I fix you something to eat? I'm sure I've got something in. I could make something and bring it over for you while we wait for your mum?"

"No!" I said, closing the door a fraction more. There was no way Mr Thurston could come inside. The moment he saw the state of the flat he would know Morag wasn't here.

He held his hands up again. "No worries. If you're concerned about me coming in, you're welcome to come over to mine. It's only across the hall. Do you have a phone? You can text your mum and let her know where you are. Or you can give me her number?"

I considered my options. I *was* hungry, and my stomach had made sure that was clear. Plus, I wasn't sure I could face another night of cereal or dry bread or broken-up biscuits scraped from the bottom of the tin.

I glanced behind me into the flat. It was quiet, dark, lonely.

"OK," I said. "I'll text her now."

"Great!" Kingsley nodded. "Make sure you let your mum know it's flat nine. She can come and join us if she likes."

I took out Morag's phone and pretended to type a message, which I then deleted. Then I grabbed my keys and followed him.

Even though it was only across the hallway, Kingsley's flat felt like it could have been miles away from ours. As soon as he unlocked his door, a wave of warmth washed over me, as though I was stepping off a plane into a hot country like Spain or somewhere. Not that I'd ever been to a place like that. He must have spent a lot of money on the heating bill. I couldn't wait to tell Morag all about it.

I stood there on the doormat, taking it all in, while Kingsley darted around, flicking on lights in every corner of the living room.

It was the same layout as our flat, but it looked totally different. Everything was smart and modern, a bit like the houses you see on magazine covers and on those house-selling shows Morag liked to watch.

There were these low grey sofas that were like furniture from the future, and a giant silver telly screen that covered almost half of the living-room wall. The walls were painted in nice colours of grey and cream, with none of the damp spots and cobwebs and bits of flaky paint that we had on ours.

Kingsley's kitchen looked space-age, with shiny drawers and cupboards with fancy metal handles. On the worktop there were all different machines with lots of buttons and screens and colours.

Best of all, in the corner of the living room was a massive fish tank that was bigger than our bathtub, all lit up from the inside. Loads of tropical fish of every colour of the rainbow were swimming around inside. The water made a quiet little bubbling sound.

"*Wow!*" I said. Maybe Kingsley was a millionaire or something.

"Take a seat, make yourself at home. Remote's on the side of the sofa there. Scroll through or you can change to the kids' channels."

"Kids' channels?" I said stupidly. We didn't have kids' channels. Not the ones you had to pay for, anyway. "I don't know how to find them."

"I can set that up for you. Come on, fella, take a seat – make yourself comfy. Are you warm enough?"

I sat down on the plump grey sofa. The cushions pulled me in like a warm hug. It was so comfy, like nothing I'd ever sat on before. Our sofa was patchy and hard, and had loads of rips in it from that time we had a kitten after Dad went.

Morag thought the kitten might cheer us up a bit, give us something to think about other than how rubbish everything was. It actually worked for a few days. We loved watching him tiptoeing around the flat and playing with the catnip toys Morag got from the pet shop. One time he clawed his way right to the top of the curtains and we couldn't believe it. I called him Socks for obvious reasons. Socks really took my mind off things … for a bit.

The only problem was that he came with fleas, which soon started jumping around on the carpet. Morag got sort of obsessed with the fleas, and that made her anxiety even worse. Morag said she'd rather have Dad back than a flea infestation, so I had a weird feeling it wasn't going to work out.

We only had Socks for two weeks before Morag said it would be best if we found him a better home, one where he could play outside. I cried so much when Morag took him away, even though he kept scratching me all the time. She gave him to someone from work.

They sent us photos of Socks for a while, of him getting bigger and friendlier. But the photos stopped when Morag lost her job.

Kingsley was flicking through a long list of channels on his super-bright telly. His telly had so many more channels than ours did. Eventually he chose a colourful cartoon about a family of racoons all fighting with each other.

"This'll do?" Kingsley asked, looking to me. "*The Racoon Bunch*? Might be a bit young for you … I don't have kids so I'm not too sure what the cool people watch these days." He laughed a little bit to himself.

"This is … amazing," I said. "I've never even seen a telly this big."

"Ah, thanks. You're a good house guest. Very easy to accommodate. Now, let me fix you some pancakes. How do you take your pancakes, neighbour? American style or European?"

I was confused. I didn't know there *were* different styles of pancakes. Nobody had ever given me a choice. I just loved pancakes and that was that.

"Normal, please," I said. "If that's OK."

"Your wish is my command. Two portions of *normal*-style pancakes coming right up!"

"I made both styles of pancakes, seeing as you couldn't decide." Kingsley put the plate down beside me. "It's about time I put some of those appliances to use."

The pancakes were like nothing I had seen before in my life. On one side of the huge plate were three stacked pancakes, each one as thick as a mattress. They were covered with a golden sauce that dripped down the sides and powdered with white sugar.

On the other side of the plate were thin pancakes, folded into neat semicircles, covered with crispy granules of sugar and lemon juice so strong it made my eyes water. These were what I called *normal* pancakes, just like we usually had on Pancake Day.

Kingsley had made himself a plate identical to mine, and he sat munching them at the other end of the sofa.

"Are they good?" he asked.

"Really good," I said through a mouthful of doughy pancake. "I really like these big ones with the sauce."

Kingsley grinned. "Ah, yes, American pancakes with maple syrup. My absolute favourite. Good with a wide variety of toppings, you know, like strawberries and crème fraiche."

"What's *crem fresh*?" I asked, wrinkling up my nose.

"It's sort of a horrible type of cream that only grown-ups like, to be honest."

"If it's so horrible, then why do you eat it on your pancakes?"

Kingsley tipped his curly head from one side to the other. "That's a great question. Probably just because the other grown-ups do it too."

"Morag says most people get really boring and stuffy when they turn into adults. She says adult life is no fun."

"Morag?" Kingsley said. "Who's Morag?"

"She's my mum. She prefers to be called Morag."

"Got it. Well, she's not wrong," he said, chewing thoughtfully. "And I guess she's had a difficult time of late."

"Did you see us in the newspapers?" I asked, not sure if I wanted to hear the answer.

"I did," he said. "I think most people have seen it, neighbour."

"Morag hit the roof."

He paused a moment before replying. "Is that why you're always wearing that suit? It makes you look like you're in a production of *Bugsy Malone*."

I stared hard at my pancakes. I didn't know what *Bugsy Malone* was, but I didn't like it when people talked about my suit.

"Sorry," he said. "I really didn't mean to be rude. It's

just you don't see many kids dressed like you around here. Let's change the subject."

"Do you have a job?" I said.

"Finance," he said. "I trade commodities. But that's not very interesting for kids. Nor for adults, come to think of it. I spend most of my time staring at computer screens like a robot, waiting until home time."

I didn't know what *finance* or *commodities* meant at all. But looking around Kingsley's flat I could tell that commodities was an amazing job. Maybe Morag should do commodities.

"Listen, neighbour," Kingsley said, clearing away my empty plate. "I don't want to be nosy. But I do hear things, you know. Shouting. Loud music at night. All that business in the papers can't be fun. If there's anything I can do … well, you know where I live, OK? Don't be afraid to knock."

"OK." I didn't think I would knock. But you never knew. After all, Kingsley did make good pancakes.

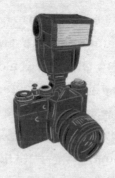

CHAPTER 30

BANG, BANG, BANG!

I woke up with a jolt in Morag's bed. My eyes were gritty with sleep, and my cheek was stuck to the pillow.

The digital alarm clock on the bedside cabinet showed the time: 07:01. I'd slept all night, stuffed full of pancakes, warmed through to my bones by Kingsley's central heating.

BANG, BANG, BANG again at the door. It wasn't the same gentle knock as Kingsley's.

Even though I had pins and needles in my legs from sleeping funny, and my head was still foggy with sleep, I pushed off the heavy covers and stumbled out of the room. Morag was back!

I threw the door open, barely containing my spreading grin. I flung my arms out wide knowing that everything would be OK and I would forgive her in an instant for running away.

"Happy Monday, matey. How's it all going?"

My heart dropped all the way down to Australia. A lanky man was standing there. He had orange, tanned skin and slicked-back hair. He was wearing a too-tight grey suit that looked uncomfortable.

I stepped back. "Who are you?"

"Main door was open – hope you don't mind. I think we've spoken on the phone once or twice. My name's Jack Morley. I'm a reporter for the *Daily News*. Just woken up, have you?" He looked at my mop of hair and grimaced.

"What do *you* want?" I asked, flattening my hair.

"I brought you these." He held out a slightly greasy paper bag that smelled like it had warm pastries inside. "Almond croissant take your fancy? There's a vanilla slice as well. Might be a bit mushed up now though."

"No thanks," I said, eyeing the bag. "I don't take food from strangers."

"Well, we both know that's not true, don't we?" He looked proper pleased with himself for that one.

Morag would have called him a *right piece of work* if she was there.

"What do you want?" I wedged my foot behind the door.

"Any sign of your mum yet, Solo? I'd like to chat with her about that interview."

"Morag's not interested in your stupid story, and neither am I!"

"Any chance she can come to the door and tell me that herself?" He peered behind me and into the flat. "And if she can't, well, that's a whole other story, if you catch my drift."

"What are you on about?"

"*Funeral Mum Missing* – quite the headline, don't you think? Even better: *Dearly Departed: Funeral Mum on the Loose.* Or we could go with a serious missing-person angle."

"You can't do that," I snapped. "She's here. She was just at the shops."

"Is that so?" He raised his eyebrows and knocked on the open door. "Ms Walker?" he bellowed into the flat. "Morag Walker, are you there? It's Jack Morley from the *Daily News*. Care for a quick chat?"

There was nothing but silence, obviously.

"You should tell the police if you don't know where

she is," he said. "Seriously. You need some help here."

Why was everyone always telling me to ask for help? It was embarrassing. I had everything under control.

"Catch you later, Solo. And I mean it – tell the police. Or I might have to."

Jack turned away on the heel of his pointy black shoe before turning back and tossing the bag of pastries into my hands. "Take these, for your trouble. Look after yourself, yeah?"

I slammed the door, trembling. I may or may not have eaten the pastries.

I paced around the flat for the next hour. The last thing we needed was more news stories about Morag. More appearances on that mean telly show. More nasty comments online.

If news got out that Morag was missing, I'd have to go and live in a home for forgotten kids. I'd have to leave school, maybe never see Chetna again. Morag would be in so much trouble that she wouldn't want to come back, even if she could.

Why didn't I have magical powers that could fix everything? I remembered a telly show I'd seen where a girl's wishes came true whenever she said them in the mirror. I knew it was silly, but I walked to the bathroom.

"M – O – R – A – G." I spelled her name out loud and spun round three times on the spot, hoping that somehow it would make her appear behind me. "M – O – R – A – G."

Nothing happened. I knew it wouldn't work, but my heart still sank when she didn't pop into the room in a puff of smoke and glitter.

I stared into the mirror at my reflection. I couldn't stand it any more. Nobody else was looking for Morag, so I would have to do it myself.

Like a tornado, I rushed to put on my school uniform, grabbed my coat and bag, and stuffed Morag's charged phone into my pocket.

Morag would be found, whether she liked it or not.

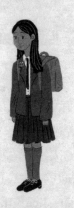

CHAPTER 31

My heart was going a thousand miles an hour. I walked as normally as I could across the playground, hoping nobody could see my chest heaving through my blazer. I wasn't planning on being at school for long, so I didn't want to be seen. I dodged sprinting kids and flying footballs.

"Watch out, Funeral Boy!" a boy yelled as he deliberately kicked the football right at my head. It only just missed me.

"Where's your mum, Solo? No funerals to crash today?"

"Only yours, when I tell Mrs Howe what you just did!" I stuck my tongue out and kept walking.

If I got into a fight, my plan would be ruined. The teachers couldn't know I was there. Especially Miss Carmichael. I walked straight to the cloakroom, leaving the boys laughing about Morag and me.

It's all water off a duck's back. That's what Morag would have said. *Water off a duck's back*.

Inside, the school was quiet. It was still early. Only the Breakfast Club kids were around. The corridors carried the delicious food smells from the canteen, but I wasn't there to eat. I had to stay focused. I had to get in and out quickly, like the time when Morag and I went to Noodle Town and left without paying. The more fuss you created, the harder it was to get away with it.

Chetna was exactly where I thought she would be. She was in Miss Cowmichael's empty classroom, sitting alone at the Cool Table and muttering to herself as she arranged her handwriting pens according to thickness.

"Solo!" she said, leaping to her feet as soon as she saw me. "I was up worrying all weekend. Is your mum back yet? I've been dying to tell someone, just dying to. But I knew that I *shouldn't* tell anyone. I just…"

"Chetna," I said, interrupting her panicked flow of words. I was worried she would talk for ever and ever and then Miss Cowmichael would come in and catch us. "Listen. I need your help with something. Have you got your phone with you today?"

Chetna started to go red with worry when I told her about Jack Morley. Then redder when I said I was going to find Morag, with her help. Her eyes went wide and she kept shaking her head.

"We should go to the police, Solo," she said. "They'll be able to help find her. Or Mrs Howe. We need to tell a grown-up. Anybody will do!"

"No!" I said. "You don't understand. If the police find Morag, she'll get in trouble and taken away. I'll be sent to a home. Same if we tell a teacher. Plus, this journalist is going to write a story about Morag being missing. It *has* to be a secret."

Chetna stared at the floor between us, her eyes shiny like glass marbles.

"But I'll get in trouble too," she said, avoiding my gaze. "My parents will kill me if I get caught truanting. I'd be grounded for the rest of my life. I'll be thirty-eight years old by the time they forgive me."

"But we won't *get* caught," I urged. "I have a secret

way out of school, and Miss Carmichael doesn't know we're here yet. We'll be back by lunchtime, I promise. I've done it loads, and nobody even notices!"

Chetna rolled her eyes. "No offence, but that's *you*, Solo. Nobody expects any different."

"Thanks for that," I said, feeling a bit hurt. But I knew she was right. "It's easy. All you have do is phone reception and say you have an appointment. Pretend to be your mum or something. That'll buy you a few hours to help me look for Morag."

"Pretend to be my mum?" Chetna looked horrified. "That's impersonating an adult. Isn't that illegal?"

I rolled my eyes. "I do it all the time. Just put on a grown-up voice; they'll never know it's you. I promise you won't get in trouble."

"How can you promise me that?"

I thought for a moment. "Even if we did get caught," I said, "you're a new kid. New kids never get in trouble for anything. You can just say you were upset about moving schools and they'll let you off!"

Chetna sighed and shook her head as if she couldn't believe what her own brain was telling her to do. "What if I did say yes. Then what?"

"We look everywhere we can until we find Morag. But I can't do it all on my own. Outside is too big and I'm only one person."

"Fine." Chetna sighed and pulled her phone from her pocket. "I can't believe I'm doing this."

I held my breath as she found the school's number online, then pressed to call it. The line began to ring.

"*Thank you for calling the reception desk. Nobody is available to take your call at the moment, so please leave a message after the tone.*"

"It's gone to voicemail," Chetna whispered, eyes wide with panic. "What do I do?"

"Leave a message!" I whispered back, giving her two thumbs up.

The line made a loud beeping sound, and Chetna cleared her throat. Her fake grown-up voice was so deep I nearly burst out laughing.

"Uh, hello there," Chetna said, staring at the floor. "I – I mean, my daughter, Chetna, won't be able to come in this morning. She has a … dentist's appointment. I'll bring her in around lunchtime. This is her mother speaking, by the way. Goodbye." She hung up the phone, grimacing.

"See," I said. "Piece of cake, wasn't it?"

"Do you *promise* we'll be back by lunchtime? I really don't want any demerits, Solo. I'm in line for another Star of the Week award."

"Already? Wow, you really are a goody two shoes."

"I know," she muttered. "I can't help it. So you promise we'll be back by lunchtime? Pinky swear?"

I hooked my little finger around hers to seal the promise. It felt weird knowing someone was on my side.

I held the escape hole in the fence open wide like a shark's jagged mouth while Chetna climbed through, careful not to catch her long hair or pristine school uniform on the edges of the wires. The morning bell had already rung, so we had to be quick.

"Thanks, Solo," she puffed, climbing to her feet and wiping the dust from the knees of her black tights. "What a convenient route."

"Cool, isn't it? I found it last year."

Chetna looked around. "It's scary out here, isn't it? Like a ghost town. No parents and teachers and cars. It's as if the world has been paused."

I smirked. Chetna had obviously never skipped school before. I was already used to quiet streets during school hours. The rest of the world changed when schoolkids weren't around. Time moved slowly, old people and cats shuffled at a snail's pace around the neighbourhood.

It meant two young kids in school uniform in the middle of the day stood out like sore thumbs. Whatever we did, wherever we went, we needed to be really careful.

"Come on, Chetna. We need to get looking if we're going to be back by lunchtime."

"Got it. Where first?"

"We'll need to split up. I'll take the bus station. You take Noodle Town."

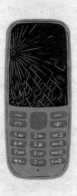

CHAPTER 32

I held Morag's cracked phone up against the glass where the ticket cashier sat, partially camouflaged by peeling stickers and sun-faded laminated signs. On the screen was a picture of Morag, one of my all-time favourites. Normally it made me smile, although today it made me sad.

The photograph was taken on one of our treat days when Morag took me out and we did fun things together. I remembered that day so well. We caught the bus into central London and went to the Natural History Museum. I saw a real human brain floating in a tank with all the nervous system dangling down like jellyfish legs.

The brain made Morag go queasy. "Come on," she'd said, trying to drag me to the next exhibit, but I was obsessed. "Let's move along before I chuck up my breakfast!"

That made me laugh so much, the thought of Morag chucking up. I remember we laughed about it the whole way through the museum, all through the fossils and the cavemen and the dinosaurs and dead butterflies stuck with pins in glass cabinets.

Afterwards Morag asked me to take a picture of her in one of the red phone boxes outside. She held the phone to her ear and grinned as if she was having the most hilarious chat with someone.

"Look at me, Solo!" she'd said, laughing. "Like a proper tourist!"

I took loads of photos, pressing the button again and again and again. When I flicked through them, they moved almost like a mini film of Morag. It was as though she was here, almost.

The ticket woman scrunched up her nose. "Nope," she huffed. "Doesn't ring a bell."

"Are you sure? She comes here all the time. Normally dressed in black, like she's going to a funeral."

She put on her glasses to look closer, but still said,

"Nope, sorry. I'll keep my eyes peeled though, love." She winked. "Not much gets past me. Twenty years I've been sat in this ticket booth and never missed a trick. Next!"

Then the person behind me in the queue pushed past, to get a return ticket to somewhere or other.

I opened Morag's phone and deleted a few missed calls from school, probably wondering where I was. Then I dialled Chetna's phone to check how she was doing.

"Don't worry, Solo," Chetna said. "Missing things are always in the last place you look, not the first."

"I know," I grumbled. "That's the whole problem. Anyway, any luck at Noodle Town?" I asked. "She absolutely loves it there."

"They weren't open yet, so no customers," Chetna said. "But the staff inside said they recognized her picture. They said something about an unpaid bill?"

I gulped, thinking of Morag's little black book of money she owed people. Of course Noodle Town was in there. I hadn't thought about that.

"Solo? Are you there? Hello?"

"Uh, yes." I paused. "I don't know what they're talking about. Just ignore them."

"They said they'd keep an eye out for her. So that's

a good thing! But we've only got two hours until lunch, Solo. Where next?"

"Morag loves pubs. Check any pubs in the nearby area, then let's meet at the train station before we head back to school."

"Pubs?" Chetna said, sounding nervous. "I don't think I'll be allowed in any pubs, Solo."

"Just look through the windows then," I said. "Or in the gardens."

"Got it. I'll let you know what I find. Don't be too long, Solo. If I'm caught off school grounds, I'm dead meat. Literally."

There was one more place I wanted to check before I met Chetna at the train station. The place that had been haunting the back of my mind like a beast creeping around in the shadows of the forest. The place where all this mess had started.

I boarded the bus that went past the Queen's Head. The driver didn't ask me for a ticket. He took one look at my new uniform and waved me on, thinking I had a travel card. Finally, this uniform was good for something.

I sat on the top deck, right at the front. Partly because it was my favourite place to sit, and partly because it was the best place to look out for Morag.

I scoured the streets as the bus trundled along, startling every time I saw a black leather jacket or messy brown hair. I pressed my nose against the glass to get a closer look each time, but none of them were her.

The bus stopped outside the Queen's Head. It looked much emptier than last time I was here. If only we'd never come here, this whole mess could have been avoided.

I remembered whinging outside, "*Why do we never do anything I want to do?*" I wish I'd never complained about Morag. Now I just wanted her back.

I pushed the door and went in. The pub was dark and cold.

"Can I help you, little fella?" the barman said. Then his face changed. "Oh, it's you."

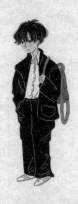

CHAPTER 33

"That all sounds pretty rubbish, if you ask me."

Alex the barman slid a free glass of cola with ice and a packet of dry roasted peanuts towards me. I chugged the cola straight down, not even needing the straw. Searching for Morag was thirsty work.

The whole Funeral Boy story had come tumbling out of me. I thought Alex would understand, since he was one of the only people who had actually seen it happen. He listened to the whole thing without speaking, just frowning a bit and shaking his head. Sometimes he would open his mouth but immediately clamp it shut. Then, when I was finished, he nodded thoughtfully.

"You're sure you haven't seen her?" I said through brain freeze.

"One hundred per cent certain. Not since that night. Not every criminal returns to the scene of the crime." He shook his head. "Not that she's a criminal. You know what I'm saying? Well, what a fiasco that turned out to be, eh? Although it was good for us."

"How do you mean?"

"Lots of punters came in, asking if this is really the pub where that whole Funeral Mum thing happened. Believe it or not, our bookings for wakes have tripled."

"Great," I said. How embarrassing.

"For what it's worth, I thought your mum was pretty funny. She definitely livened up my shift that day."

I laughed, but only out of my nose. Morag could be funny, but she could also be a total nightmare. Right now, she was leaning more towards nightmare.

"If she's gone missing, you should tell someone." Alex refilled my glass with the cool spray nozzle from under the bar. "What about your dad? Can't he do anything?"

I laughed properly then. "I haven't spoken to him in five years."

Alex rolled his eyes. "Dads, eh? Well, how about a teacher? You can't be out traipsing all over town on your own." He turned to restock the hanging cardboard rail of pork scratchings. "What are you? Eight years old?"

"I'm ten, actually."

"Ah, I see," he said a bit sarcastically. "So you're all grown up, then."

I chomped on my peanuts, grateful for the salty distraction. I noticed someone peering out of the kitchen door, holding their phone up. They saw me looking and the door swung shut suspiciously quickly.

"I should go," I said, handing my empty glass back. Morag's phone was buzzing in my pocket. It was probably Chetna, wondering where I'd got to. I scrawled Morag's number on to the back of a cardboard coaster. "Promise you'll keep an eye out for her?"

"You got it, kiddo. Keep your chin up."

Chetna was hiding behind an overflowing bin when I found her at the train station. I spotted her from across the road. She was trembling. Her eyes darted from side to side.

"Where on earth have you been? It's gone twenty past twelve! We've got less than ten minutes to get back to school before everyone will notice we're not in the lunch queue. My phone says it takes at least twenty minutes to walk there!"

"Any sign of Morag?" I asked.

Chetna ignored me. "I'm going to get in so much trouble. I'll be kicked out of Spanish club. Netball won't want me. What about choir? I haven't even done one practice yet and I'm already going to be labelled a truant."

"Snap out of it, Chetna! It's all going to be fine, I promise."

"Sorry," she panted. "I've just never been in any trouble whatsoever. I don't think I'd cope well in detention. I'm just not cut out for it."

"I've had plenty of detentions," I said. "And look at me – I'm doing all right, aren't I?"

"You don't want me to answer that honestly, do you?"

"I guess not," I said. "We should go."

"Good idea. You've really got a mind for this rule-breaking stuff, by the way."

"Thanks," I said. I knew exactly where I'd got it from.

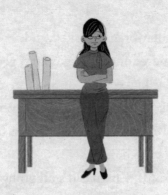

CHAPTER 34

It's surprising how fast I can run when I really try. We got back to school at 12.45 p.m. exactly, which was late, but not late enough for anyone to notice.

Nobody saw us crawling back through the escape hole, and we simply weaved ourselves into the crowd of kids running around and playing. Our class was already lining up to go inside for lunch. Panting, we joined the back of the queue.

"Chetna! Solo!" Miss Carmichael said. My stomach went icy cold. "Good to see you both. How was it at the dentist's, Chetna?"

"No fillings!" Chetna beamed, showing all her teeth. "And the dentist said my brushing technique is second to none! In fact, it got me thinking about being a dentist when I grow up."

I looked at Chetna, blown away. For such a goody-goody, she was brilliant at making up lies on the spot. It was seriously impressive, actually.

"Oh, I'm glad to hear it," Miss Carmichael replied, clearly impressed. "And, Solo – another late night, I assume? Reception have been trying to call your mum all morning."

"Sorry, Miss," I said, stifling a yawn. "I didn't sleep well. Plus, Mum's phone's been broken for ages."

"Well, you're here now – that's what counts, but it has to be noted. While I have you both," Miss Carmichael said, flipping through the sheets on her clipboard, "I don't seem to have a signed permission slip for tomorrow's trip from either of you. You won't want to miss Normley-on-Sea's stunning geographical features! Slips returned first thing, please. Or you'll be spending the day in the library."

Normley-on-Sea. Normley-on-Sea.

The name rattled around my brain. Normley-on-Sea. I'd been there. It was where the Sunset Dunes caravan park was. The place where me and Morag went on holiday every year, before she lost her job and everything became difficult. The place where we had our photo taken – me as an old-fashioned diver, Morag a sucker-covered octopus.

I felt myself fizzing with the bubbles of a new idea.

"How much is the trip, Miss?" I asked.

"Ten pounds," she said. "You can bring the cash on the day."

"We'll do that, Miss Carmichael," said Chetna.

Miss Carmichael turned away, and the lunch queue began to move.

"I can't believe we got away with that," she said. "Feels kind of exciting, being rebellious."

"Chetna," I said, "you're not going to like it, but I have another plan to find Morag."

She leaned close to me. "What? What is it?"

"Before I tell you, I need to ask if I can borrow ten pounds."

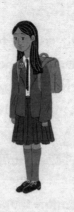

CHAPTER 35

Forging Morag's signature had always been easy.
Actually, I wondered if Morag had made it easy on
purpose. Her signature was just an *M* followed by a
squiggle. I'd been giving myself signed permission on
Morag's behalf for things since Year Two.

On Tuesday, Mrs McDonald – Katy's mum – seemed
surprised when I produced the screwed-up yellow
permission slip from my trouser pocket. We still
had to wear our school uniform on trips, because
apparently we were representing the whole school. She
ticked my name off the register and hesitated.

"And the, er…" Mrs McDonald cleared her throat.
"Have you got the ten pounds?"

"Oh, yeah, sorry. Here." I fished around and

produced an equally crinkly ten-pound note, which Chetna's parents had given her to buy snacks with. She'd told them ten pounds was the recommended amount. She was getting good at lying.

"Brilliant," said Mrs McDonald. "OK. Hop on! So glad you could join us, Solo. Don't forget to collect your map from the pile at the front of the coach!"

I took a map from the top of the pile and climbed onboard.

The coach smelled of dust and packed lunches. Chetna had saved a seat for me in the middle. It was far enough away from Kai Bailey and his gang who had taken up the entire back row, thinking it made them look tough.

"Did it work? With the permission slip?" Chetna asked.

I winked. "Always does. Thanks for the tenner, by the way. I promise I'll give it back as soon as I can."

"Don't worry about it." Chetna checked over her shoulders to make sure nobody was listening. "Tell me the plan again. I need to make sure I have everything straight."

"OK. When we're walking around Normley-on-Sea, you and me sneak off. We check Morag's favourite places, and then we re-join everybody just before the coach brings us home at five o'clock."

Chetna seemed scared. "This feels risky, Solo. *Really* risky."

"It is," I said. "But it's going to be fine. We got away with it yesterday, didn't we?"

Chetna nodded, but she looked sick and pale, even though the coach wasn't moving yet.

"What if we don't?" she whispered. "Make it back in time, that is."

"Well, then I guess we'll be sleeping on the dodgems for the night."

Chetna gasped, horrified. "Don't say that."

"I'm joking," I said. "There's always the train."

"Right then, everybody!" Miss Carmichael stood at the front of the coach, holding a microphone. "Who's ready to see some real-life coastal erosion? Give me a cheer!"

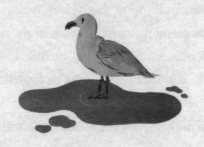

CHAPTER 36

The air in Normley-on-Sea was ice cold. As soon as we got off the coach, the wind rushed in and cut right through my new uniform. My skin went into a rash of goosebumps. I clenched my teeth, trying not to shiver.

"Why is it so c-c-cold?" Chetna said through chattering teeth, as the wind flung her black hair around her head like a curtain being whipped back and forth.

I didn't know what to say. I'd imagined Normley-on-Sea to be hot and sunny like it was the last time Morag and I had visited. I thought the air would smell like the sea and hot sugared doughnuts and coconut-flavoured sun cream. I thought I'd hear families laughing, and the music of the ice-cream van selling 99 Flake ice creams. I thought I'd hear fairground rides, fruit machines spinning, sizzling chip friers.

Instead, everything was grey, damp and deserted. Thick black clouds hung heavy in the sky like wet bed sheets on the washing line. The few people milling around were old and miserable-looking. They were wrapped up tight in padded coats, woolly hats and scarves. Across the car park, a seagull regurgitated a chewed-up chip into a puddle.

This wasn't the Normley-on-Sea that I remembered, where I'd built sandcastles, been on my first roller coaster and had my photo taken in an old-fashioned metal diving suit with Morag. It was as though everyone had forgotten about Normley-on-Sea and left it behind, turning it into a ghost town.

It wasn't the Normley-on-Sea where Morag went paddling and accidentally went so deep that she was waist high in the water, swimming around in her black clothes, not caring that people were looking. Where Morag had forced me to dance with her to the music the buskers played on their penny whistles – she'd laughed hysterically the whole time while I tried to slip out of her arms.

If Morag was here, she wouldn't recognize this

gloomy, sad version of Normley-on-Sea at all. Her Big
Bad Reds would probably be worse than ever before.

"OK then, class," Miss Carmichael shouted. "We'll
begin by making our way to some coastal cottages,
whose foundations are slowly creeping closer to the
water's edge, thanks to erosion. The residents have
kindly agreed to let us in their gardens, so I want you
on your best behaviour…"

Mrs McDonald began counting us in pairs. This
was our moment, before she counted me and Chetna.
And that's when I saw that Mrs McDonald had left
the register on top of her bag, in front of the coach.
I quickly reached over and stuffed the sheet into my
trouser pocket. How would they notice we were gone
without the register?

"Now," I whispered to Chetna, jerking my head
towards an alleyway that cut away from the car park.

"Now?" She looked startled. "I thought we would at
least get to see a *bit* of the coastal erosion!"

"No time!"

I grabbed Chetna's sleeve and we darted down the
alley. We hid until the sound of chatter faded, and all
we could hear was whistling wind and the crashing
of the sea.

"What will we do with Morag, even if we do find

her?" Chetna asked. "Won't it be a bit weird if your mum turns up halfway through the trip and rides the coach home with us?"

"We'll make something up. We'll say I got homesick and she had to come and find me or something. I don't care if it makes me look stupid."

"Do you really think she'll be here, Solo? It's a bit…" She looked around, searching for the right word. "Dreary, isn't it?"

"Well, sorry about that," I said, offended. "Not everyone can afford to go to Disney World Florida on holiday every year. This is where we always go, Morag and me. We really like it here."

Chetna went red. "You know I didn't mean it like that, Solo. I'm sure it's lovely in the summer."

"It's just the weather," I said. "It's not normally like this, honestly. You'll have to trust me. It's Morag's favourite place in the whole world. I should have thought of it sooner."

"OK, OK, I believe you," she said, trying to calm her shivering. "So where do we start?"

I dragged Chetna to the end of the alley, which overlooked the whole of Normley-on-Sea. There were rows of grey houses leading to a long, sandy beach, with loads of tourist attractions on the beachfront – and at the far end was Sunset Dunes caravan park.

"There." I pointed towards the beachfront. "Morag loves it down there. We'll start with the arcade, then the promenade, then the Sea View Cafe."

The sea was churning like mucky washing-machine water. The palm trees that usually looked so tropical seemed sad, their leaves faded brown and drooping.

"If she's not there," I added, "we'll try the caravan park. She might be tucked up in a caravan, watching the telly with a nice cup of tea."

Or a nice cup of something else, I thought.

With that, we headed out into the wind.

Chetna was quiet for a while. Then she said, "Just so you know, I've never actually been to Disney World Florida. I object to it. My sister loves movies about princesses and fairies, but I think they give people unrealistic expectations and increase pressure for real life to be some sort of fairy tale, when it isn't."

I rolled my eyes. "All right, Chetna. Whatever you say."

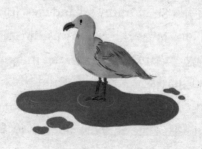

CHAPTER 37

The first place we searched was the arcade. It had that stale smell that abandoned places have: a weird mixture of dust and central heating, which went straight up my nostrils. It was dark, with only the occasional flashing golden lights coming from the displays on the fruit machines and 2p coin pushers.

Last time I'd visited, it was packed full of tourists. The sounds of coins cascading and machines whirring had almost deafened me. People had been playing racing games, shooting games, taking long run-ups to punch the boxing machine as hard as they could.

Morag and I had won reels and reels of paper tickets, so many that I had to wrap them round both arms like a mummy's bandages just to keep track of them. Splat the Snail was our strong suit, and we played again and again, me imagining each popping-up snail was Kai Bailey and the Cool Table lot. Over the week, Morag and I had got so good at splatting snails that we even got on to the leader board with a first-place high score. I remembered Morag typing in our names in capitals – SOLOMORAG because there wasn't enough space to put "and" in the middle.

Turned out even our hundreds of winning tickets was only enough for a pencil and eraser, but they were still the only things I'd ever won, so I loved them.

Now nobody was here, and the arcade games were silent. In fact, there were barely any signs of life. No music, no staff. No spools of prize tickets printing out all over the floor. Huge piles of cuddly toys were lying at the bottom of the claw-grabbing games, their open eyes peering out at us, almost begging to be picked.

"Creepy in here, isn't it?" I said.

"Yeah," Chetna said, gawping. "It's like something from a horror film." She glanced at me. "I don't like horror films, Solo."

As she said that, she stepped back and accidentally

pushed a button on one of the machines. It instantly sprang to life in an explosion of music and lights, which sent chills of shock coursing through my body.

I spun round to find a big glass box with the robotic head and shoulders of a man trapped inside. He was dressed in a turban decorated with gemstones and jewels, and a fancy-looking silk jacket. He started moving, jerkily beckoning us closer with his plastic hands.

"*May your destiny be unshrouded,*" the machine blared in a booming voice. "*To find what it is you are seeking, insert only two one-pound coins.*"

Chetna screamed, which scared me even more. I stumbled and tripped into a fruit machine, another of Morag's favourites, which also whirred to life. Dials started spinning randomly on their own, bells started dinging, lights started flashing.

"*Unlock the mystery of your future,*" the robot man in the glass box continued, his voice even louder now. "*Search no longer, your fortune awaits. Insert only two one-pound coins to experience the wisdom of the legendary great-great-gr-gr—*"

The robot man started jolting and jerking, just like when Morag's CDs got scratched and played the same snippet of music over and over again.

"What's happening?" Chetna yelled.

"I don't know!" I yelled back. "How do we make it stop?"

"*Great-gr-gr-great-great—*" The machine kept glitching and stuttering. "*The lege-lege-legendary—*"

The twitching and jerking became so rapid that I thought the robot man might burst through the glass and escape. Sparks began to emerge from the joints where his fake arms met his shoulders, and his head started banging back and forth with a horrible metallic *clunk, clunk, clunk.*

Then, with a worrying hiss, a slow stream of grey smoke snaked up from somewhere deep inside his open mouth. The music stopped. Silence crept in.

Chetna exhaled slowly. "Thank goodness. That scared the living daylights out of me." She fake-laughed to hide her panic, a hand pressed against her chest as if it was keeping her heart inside.

I laughed too, but my arms and legs felt so wobbly I was sure I would collapse to the floor like a pile of clothes with nobody inside them.

"Must be some sort of fortune-telling machine," Chetna said, strolling over to the sparking robot. "If only we actually had two one-pound coins. Maybe he could help us find Morag."

"Is somebody there?" a woman's voice called out from the back of the arcade. "Is somebody messing with my fortune teller?"

Chetna turned to me, her eyes wide and white as plates. "Hide!"

We glanced around, willing some hidey-hole to appear – and there it was. A novelty photo booth, the kind that did pencil-effect portraits and backgrounds like the Eiffel Tower, to make it look like you'd been abroad when you hadn't. We dashed inside the little booth and pulled the red velvet curtain across us.

"Did you not read the laminated sign? It says he's out of order," the voice continued. She sounded angry – and stepping closer with each word. "Blimmin' manufacturers," she muttered to herself. "They were meant to come out last week to check him over. It's a fire hazard."

Chetna tapped me on the arm, then pointed down. "Legs!"

I realized with horror that the velvet curtain was only covering the top halves of our bodies. Our trousers and shoes were clearly visible to anyone on the outside.

"Get on here!" I whispered.

We tried to crouch on top of the tiny plastic stool

inside, which was hardly big enough for one person to sit on, let alone two people to stand on. Our feet barely fitted on its slippery surface, and it creaked under our weight.

"Is someone there?" The woman was closer now, so close I was convinced she would hear us breathing. She went on muttering angrily: "I told them, out of warranty or not, I can't have a rogue machine spitting sparks under my roof. I said, he'll scare off the punters. Not that there are any punters at this time of year, anyway."

My shoes were starting to slip, and I tried to grip on to the walls with my fingertips. Chetna's feet were slipping too. Without warning, the stool dropped straight to the floor with a deafening *clunk*. Chetna and I lay at the bottom of the booth in an embarrassing tangle. We should have remembered that photo-booth stools could be adjusted.

"Ouch," Chetna groaned, rubbing her head. "Well, that worked well."

"There you are!" A hand pulled back the velvet curtain and a woman peered down at us. "I was starting to think I was hearing things. Wouldn't be the first time! Sorry if my robotic oracle gave you a bit of a fright. I'm Beryl – this is my arcade."

I breathed a sigh of relief. Beryl didn't seem angry. In fact, she was smiling, holding out two wrinkled hands with painted gold nails to help us.

"We don't get many folk in here at this time of year," she said, pulling us up. "I was thinking maybe we ought to just board everything up until spring, cut my losses. But here you are! Customers at last!"

Chetna and I patted cobwebs from our clothes.

"Sorry about that," Chetna said, glancing at the smouldering robotic fortune teller. "I leaned on it by accident and he just started ... well, doing that."

"No bother." Beryl shrugged. "He's been on the blink for ages. That said, spitting sparks and emitting toxic smoke is new. Hey, maybe it's a bad omen!" She winked and laughed a naughty cackling laugh that reminded me of Morag.

"That's a relief." Chetna exhaled, smiling a bit. "I thought I'd broken him."

"Oh no, he's useless anyway." Beryl stared at the fortune-telling machine. "Always gives the same advice: *Don't count on it.* I always think, don't count on *what*?" She gave her sandpapery laugh again.

Chetna and I looked at each other and laughed cautiously too.

"So what can I do for you?" Beryl said. "We've got

plenty of games suitable for kids over there. We've got dance machines, Shoot-a-Hoop, you name it. Strictly over-eighteens only on the fruit machines though."

"Err, we're not here to play games, I'm afraid," I said, finding my voice. I fished around in my pocket and produced Morag's cracked mobile phone. "We're looking for someone. She used to like coming here, so we thought we'd check if she'd visited."

"OK, let old Beryl take a look-see," she said, reaching out for the phone. "But as I told you, the town's dead as a dodo this time of year."

I handed Beryl the phone, and she slid a thick pair of glasses down from her grey head of hair and on to her nose. She squinted at the photo and pinched at the screen with two fingers to zoom in.

"Hmmm," she said, before giving it back. "She's familiar, but then again I've seen a lot of faces in my time here. Thirty-two years I've owned this place."

"She would have visited in the last week," I explained. "She might even still be in Normley."

"Oh, I see. Can't say I've noticed her, I'm afraid."

I groaned. "Are you sure? This was one of her favourite places. We always used to play Splat the Snail. We got the high score on the leader board and everything!"

Beryl nodded slowly, impressed. "A high score on

Splat the Snail is no mean feat. You must be quite deft with a rubber mallet."

"Does anyone else work here?" asked Chetna.

"Only my husband, Bill, during the off season, and he spends half the time sleeping in the back office. I tell him, the games won't maintain themselves, but he's a cantankerous old— Actually, never mind that. Who is she, this woman?"

Chetna went to reply, but I shot her a warning glance. We couldn't tell Beryl that Morag was my mum, or she would start asking more questions, maybe even tell the police. Questions always led to trouble.

"Just someone we know," I said, hating myself for saying that about Morag. "We haven't seen her in a while."

"OK, well…" Beryl adjusted the many jangly silver bracelets that decorated her arms. "I'll keep an eye out. Like I said, Normley-on-Sea's a ghost town about now. You'll have better luck in April, at half-term – that's when it all comes alive again."

"OK, thanks." I turned and started to leave the arcade, my feet scuffing the carpet. I couldn't wait until April. April was ages away. Morag could be on the other side of the world by then.

"Thanks for helping us up," Chetna said, waving

goodbye. "And sorry about the fortune-teller thing."

"No bother at all, sweetheart," Beryl called after us. "Good luck!"

"Don't worry, Solo," Chetna said, catching up to me. "There're still plenty of places to look."

I stopped by the Splat the Snail machine where Morag and me had spent so many 50p coins and hours. Without thinking, I hit the start button with a hollow *thwack*, and the game quietly whirred to life. Our names were still there on the digital leader board: SOLOMORAG. Still undefeated. My eyes stung with the memory.

INSERT 50P NOW scrolled across the little screen, nudging our names away with each new letter that appeared. I sighed and walked away.

"Solo, look!" Chetna whacked the start button again, and the leader board returned to the screen.

"What?" I said.

"Come here and properly *look*!"

I joined her at Splat the Snail and read the screen. I had to blink and blink again, because I couldn't believe what was written there in blocky digital text. In fourth place, among the other names on the leader board, the screen flashed MORAG.

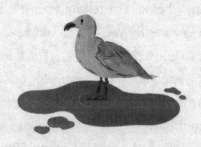

CHAPTER 38

"She's here!" I said, bursting on to the rainy promenade. The sea was all brown and topped with a creamy white foam like a horrible cappuccino. "She has to be here!"

"She *might* be here," Chetna said. "Let's not get too ahead of ourselves just yet."

"But you saw it? Right there on the screen. It said *Morag*! Splat the Snail was always our favourite arcade game. She's brilliant at it!"

"What if it's somebody else? It could be another Morag who also happens to play Splat the Snail…"

"How many people do you know called Morag?"

"Well, none," said Chetna. "OK, I see your point. But it doesn't necessarily mean—"

"It's her, Chetna. I'm telling you, it's her. Maybe she's leaving clues for me. She would have known I'd come here to find her and that I'd go on Splat the Snail. She's here waiting for me!"

"Solo…"

But I could barely hear what Chetna was saying. I felt as though I'd been charged up with the power of a hundred batteries. I had to look at every single person on the promenade twice, then again, to check whether they were Morag in disguise.

"Hello! Have you seen this woman?" I blurted, holding Morag's phone out to an old grey man in a beige anorak, startling him as he shuffled past. He shook his head without even looking and skulked away into the drizzle.

Next, I ran up to an old lady who was sitting alone on a covered bench, huddling away from the freezing wind and pelting-sideways rain.

"Sorry to bother you," I panted. "Have you seen this woman?"

"She ain't here. Look around you – nobody's here." She grimaced, turning away from Morag's photograph. "You tourists stole the heart out of this town… Now look at it! It's nothing but an empty shell of what it used to be."

"Come on, Solo." Chetna grabbed me by the back of my blazer and dragged me away to another sheltered bench further down the promenade. "You're drawing too much attention to yourself."

"I don't care! I'll speak to every single person in Normley-on-Sea if I have to! Somebody must have seen her!"

"We need to be more specific about our objectives, Solo. We're only here for a day, remember. We need to use our time efficiently."

I rolled my eyes right the way back so I could practically see my brain. It sounded exactly like something Miss Carmichael would say.

"You should be a teacher when you're older, you know." I didn't mean it as a nice thing. "You sound like one already."

"Thank you." Chetna beamed, peeling wet strands of hair from her face. "I've been considering it, actually. Now we need to decide where next."

It was easy to see that Morag was not inside the Sea View Cafe, having a nice hot cup of tea like I'd imagined. All the windows and doors had been boarded up with rotting planks. The words *BACK IN SPRING* had been sprayed on to the wood in scruffy black letters.

Last time I'd been there, we'd queued for twenty-five minutes for the best fish and chips I'd ever had in my life. Morag had hers drenched in so much vinegar it hurt my eyes to sit next to her. Afterwards, we queued again to get ice creams, and mine melted all over my hands in sticky streaks. Morag had to tell me which part to lick next to stop the mess completely engulfing my arm.

I peered through the gaps in the boards and into the dark cafe. It was silent and dusty. The chairs were stacked up on the tables, just like we did at the end of school days.

The glass cabinets didn't have any cakes or sausage rolls inside, and the ice-cream fridge was completely empty. Only the rounded metal ice-cream scoops remained, standing upright in an empty pint glass.

Chetna sighed and pressed up against the boards to avoid the rain. "Now what?"

Huge drips of water were trickling down her nose and splashing on to her shoes. We had walked for half an hour against sheets of salty rain to find the Sea View Cafe. My trousers were clinging tight to my skin, and my fingers were going wrinkly, like I'd been in the bath too long.

"I wonder if everyone else is as wet as we are," Chetna said. "And whether the erosion was interesting. I hope we don't have to do any homework about it, when we haven't even *seen* the effects of coastal erosion first-hand."

I wasn't really listening to her. I was too busy scouring for clues for Morag.

"I don't know how I'm going to explain why I'm soaking wet to my parents," she continued. "Rain is one thing, but this is something else. They'll just know I've been up to no good. I'll have to say I fell in a pond or something. But they'll never believe that."

I blinked away the trickles of rain that were slipping down from my eyebrows. *Where are you, Morag?*

"Maybe we could find some mud or algae and just smear it into my hair a bit." Chetna grimaced. "That would make it a bit more believable. Even better, I could take a quick dip in an actual pond, if we see one. At least I would smell authentic. But the amphibians… I can't." She shook her head as if shaking away the idea.

"Don't worry about that," I said, still peering into the empty cafe, hoping for signs of life. "There're heaters on the coach. I've dried clothes on buses loads of times. You'll just be damp by the time we get home, not soaked." I straightened up. "Only Sunset Dunes left now. It's the only other place I can think of."

We walked on through the sheets of rain.

Past the distant end of the promenade, tucked behind the lumpy, grass-covered dunes, was Sunset Dunes caravan park. It was a series of green-and-white caravans, all placed in rows at funny angles going up a hill. Droopy palm trees lined the outside, and the fence was decorated with multicoloured fairy lights, which weren't switched on.

Morag and I loved the cosy caravans, each with its own small kitchen and the sofa that was attached to the wall. We loved the games and the amusements and the singers performing every night. Plus, it was right next to the beach for paddling.

Even when it rained, we loved the tinny sound of the raindrops falling on the caravan roof. It was snug, like we were in a nest. Still, it seemed unlikely she would be there when everything was shut and it rained the whole time.

Please be there, Morag. I couldn't think of *anywhere* else.

There was an unofficial path that led directly from

the beach and into the heart of Sunset Dunes, so we didn't have to go through the main entrance. Morag and I used that path all the time on holiday, stepping over brambles and stones in our bare sandy feet on the way to the beach, carrying our buckets and spades and flip-flops in our arms.

Now the brambles had grown to twice the height, and the ground was slippery with rain and slugs. Every time I picked my way through another prickly bramble bush, the branches would swing back and hit Chetna, which made the trek take twice as long as usual.

Eventually we emerged from the bushes in front of the main building of Sunset Dunes. It was called the Pavilion. The Pavilion was where the entertainment happened – all the bingo and performances, and a loud disco every night. Just like everything else in Normley-on-Sea, it looked forgotten in the winter, not how I remembered it at all. The roof was caked in greenish-white seagull poo, and the P from the Pavilion sign was missing.

This weird version of the Pavilion looked nothing like the place where Morag sang "Money, Money, Money" at karaoke and got a standing ovation from the whole audience. Or where I'd played skittles with some kids from another family who all had curly ginger hair. I probably would have made proper friends with them if they hadn't had to go back to Liverpool the next morning. It didn't feel like that Pavilion at all.

I walked up to the door and looked for a sign of life. A sun-faded poster was tacked on to the inside of the window, showing last summer's performance schedule. Mickey McKee had been the headline act. His photograph was pointing right at me, grinning with glinting white teeth, like he was just so happy. He was dressed in a sparkly gold jacket and pointy dancing shoes. **SHOW TUNES FOR ALL AGES!** screamed the poster.

"It doesn't look very open, Solo," Chetna said, staring into the reception.

"Some people live here all year round," I said. "Morag told me that."

We started walking again through the caravan park, and my legs felt heavy. The bottoms of my feet were numb, as if they were telling me to stop, but I couldn't. Not until we saw some sign of Morag.

"Morag?" I cried out every so often. "Morag?"

Only seagulls bothered to reply. They were circling over us, probably waiting for us to drop a chip. Not that we had any.

Each part of Sunset Dunes had its own name, as if each strip of metal caravans was a street. We started on Sunset Walk, then turned right into Albatross Way. Each caravan was as dark and still as the Pavilion had been, with most of the sofas and dining tables covered in plastic to protect them against the dust and damp.

We trudged past the playground area where Morag and I had once swung on the monkey bars until the palms of our hands were dry and stinging. Morag was loads better at it than me, but then again she could almost touch the ground with her feet, so it was easier for her.

We saw the squishy tiled area where I'd ridden my first-ever hoverboard, propped up by one of the people who worked at Sunset Dunes. It had only taken me five minutes to get the hang of it and, before I knew it, I was whizzing all over the place. Morag was rubbish and kept falling over. I guess we were even, then.

On Starfish Crescent, the caravans became much fancier. They were surrounded by wooden decking that was topped with fake plastic grass and deckchairs for sunbathing. They had widescreen tellies with all the channels, instead of the tiny box ones. They also had proper sofas that weren't fixed on to the walls, and kitchens twice the size of what we had at home. These caravans were called "platinum", and Morag always said we would stay in one next time we came, when she had saved up the money.

I supposed there wouldn't be a next time any more, not since the whole funeral thing and Morag going missing. Morag would never have the money to go on holiday again without a job, and she would never get one now. I didn't want to go with anyone except her. I scuffed my feet as we walked on. It was starting to get dark.

"Morag?" I yelled, my voice starting to feel dry. "Are you here?"

The only response was the sound of my own voice echoing around the silent park. There was no point in screaming Morag's name any more. She wasn't here. Nobody was here but us.

"Let's just go," I said. Suddenly I felt too tired, too cold, too numb to carry on. "She isn't here. Let's just go back to the coach."

"Solo—" Chetna stopped dead in her tracks and grabbed my arm. "Look. Over there."

"What?" I said, but I saw instantly what Chetna meant. Chills went down my spine.

Inside the very last caravan on Starfish Crescent, right before the pavement became the back of the sand dunes, a light was shining. It looked like the light of a telly, all blue and dark colours shifting and reflecting into the living-room area.

"Is someone in there?" said Chetna.

"I have no idea." I noticed, kind of embarrassed, that I was clinging on to Chetna's sleeve. She didn't shrug my hand away. "What do we do?"

"Well, I guess we find out if it's her and take it from there," she replied. "If you're ready, that is?"

We started walking towards the caravan and my heart began to tick so hard I could feel the vibration all through my body. Maybe it really was Morag inside the caravan. After everything, after running away with Chetna, sneaking away from the trip, getting rained on and shouted at and attacked by a broken fortune-telling machine … maybe we'd found her.

"Wait," I said, pulling Chetna to a halt. "If it is really her, what am I supposed to say? What if she doesn't want to come home?"

She rubbed my elbow. "Whatever you feel like saying will be the right thing to say, Solo."

"What if she's not happy to see me? What if she bites our heads off for finding her hiding place? She hates it when I go behind her back."

"At least you'll know where she is, and we could

finally tell someone," said Chetna. "Someone who can help, like a *teacher*. Which, frankly, is what we should have done right at the beginning of this mess."

"Maybe we should leave it," I said, turning round. "This was a stupid idea anyway. She'll come home when she wants to, I know she will. She's always—"

"No, Solo!" Chetna grabbed my arm and pulled me back to face her. She was breathing hard. "I have not broken every rule known to civilized society just for you to walk away at the very last moment. You *have* to go in there and talk to her."

"No!" I yanked my arm back, harder than I meant to. "Get off me, Chetna! I'm not going in. You can't tell me what to do!"

"Fine," Chetna snapped. "If you won't go in and face her, then I will! I'll tell her that you've been looking everywhere for her, but at the last second you decided you couldn't even be bothered to—"

"No!"

"Is somebody there?" a voice called into the dusk. Somebody had opened one of the windows of the caravan. A shadow was leaning out, silhouetted by the light of the telly. "Hello? This is private property, you know!"

Chetna and I stopped dead.

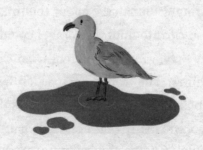

CHAPTER 39

In the caravan kitchenette, the singer Mickey McKee whistled as he stirred hot-chocolate powder, milk and hot water into two mugs for Chetna and me. He looked totally different from his poster. Rather than his gleaming gold jacket, he wore baggy jogging bottoms, a red football top, and odd flip-flops on his feet. His skin wasn't as orange as it was on his poster, but his teeth were still bright, shining white.

None of that mattered though. He wasn't Morag.

Chetna kept shifting in her seat and looking at me as if she wanted to say something, but I couldn't read her mind.

What? I mouthed.

She tapped her wrist, pointing at a watch she wasn't

even wearing. I didn't care about the time, not now. We were so close to finding Morag, I could feel it.

Mickey's caravan was different from the others at Sunset Dunes. The walls were packed with framed photographs of pop stars and rock stars. It was only when I looked closely that I realized half the photos were of him, performing on stage in various wigs and costumes. A smoky incense stick was burning in the corner, and above the dining table was a mirror surrounded by light bulbs, as if we were backstage at a theatre or something.

"Well, I haven't had a visitor here in a long while," he said. His accent was from up north or something. "Not many outsiders in Normley this time of year, I must say."

"Yeah," I said. "I usually come here every summer with my mum. It's quite … different now."

"You can say that again, kid. The whole town goes into hibernation mode once summer's over. I feel like a pet tortoise, trapped inside a shell for six months." He banged on his caravan wall, which made a metallic clank. "Who is this Morag woman again?"

"She's our scout leader," Chetna said out of nowhere. "But she hasn't been at our scout meetings for weeks. We're all searching for her today."

"Really, scout leader, you say?" Mickey raised an eyebrow as if he didn't believe us, but he didn't say anything. "You say she loves Sunset Dunes, eh? Is she a regular?"

"Yeah." I nodded. "It's her favourite place ever. She won the karaoke competition here once. Got a standing ovation and everything."

Mickey nodded slowly. "The crowds are superb here at Sunset. Quite receptive, I find."

He placed the two mugs in front of us, and we immediately picked them up to warm our hands.

"Show me again," he said, motioning to Morag's phone.

"Sure." I held the phone out so Mickey could see.

"Nope, sorry," he said. "Don't know her. She looks like a good laugh though."

"She is," I said. "Most of the time."

"Is there anyone else here who might have seen her?" Chetna said between sips of hot chocolate. "We are fairly sure she's been here in Normley-on-Sea in the last few days."

Mickey McKee chuckled and shook his head. "No, love – after summer, I'm jack of all trades. Groundskeeper, maintenance man, cleaner, you name it. Only thing I'm not doing is treading that Pavilion stage, belting my show-tunes repertoire. If anyone had been here, I would know."

"I see," Chetna said. "Thank you for the hot chocolate. It's lovely."

"No problem. You both look absolutely freezing. Did the scouts not give you any proper winter coats? They should have known Normley's famed for its horizontal rain and gale-force winds this time of year. So much for always being prepared!" Mickey wheezed at his own joke, but I didn't get it.

"We left our bags on the coach," Chetna said. "By accident."

Mickey nodded. "I see. Where's the rest of your troop, then?"

"Checking other parts of Normley," replied Chetna. "You know, all the sights. Speaking of which, we should probably get going, Solo. We don't want them to worry about us." She glared at me as she said that.

"Err, yeah," I said, even though I didn't want to put down my hot chocolate. Mickey had put too much chocolate powder in mine, so it was nice and thick.

"Will you keep an eye out?" I asked him. "If you see her, tell her Solo came looking for her."

"Solo," Mickey said, trying the name out. "Odd choice for a name, isn't it? Definitely unique though. Has a certain star quality."

"Thanks," I said. I didn't want to be a star. I only wanted to find Morag. "My mum chose it."

"We should *really* get going," Chetna said again, sounding more urgent now.

Mickey was staring at me intensely over his steaming mug. "I recognize that name, Solo, come to think of it."

"Really?" I laughed nervously. "I'm not sure why that would be."

Mickey rummaged down the side of his armchair and produced a rolled-up copy of *The Herald*. My stomach lurched as he unfurled it.

"Isn't this you?" he said, pointing to the photo on the front page. The photo that had started all this. "And isn't that … her?" His eyes widened as he realized the truth. Funeral Boy was sitting in *his* caravan.

"No," I said. "I don't even know what that is."

"You're not scouts," he said slowly, looking from Chetna to me. "You're scammers. I've read all about you in the papers, you know. Is she here too, that Funeral Mum?"

255

"No!" I protested. "I promise we're not trying to—"

"Nobody pulls a fast one on old Mickey McKee. I'm calling the authorities right away. How did you even get on site? We've had the main entrance barricaded for weeks now."

"We came through the beach path," I said. "We didn't mean to—"

"Hello, site security?" Mickey said into his phone. "Bit of a weird one, but I've got two kids here, apparently looking for some missing woman. One's that Funeral Boy, off the news. All feels a bit funny, if you ask me."

"Run, Solo!" Suddenly Chetna was on her feet, halfway out of the caravan door before I even had time to register her instruction.

I got to my feet, and so did Mickey McKee.

"No, no, no you don't!" He held his palms out to me. "You wait here. The security guards will take care of you, don't you worry."

I looked between Mickey and the open door. Sheets of rain were lashing the ground. I bolted, knocking my hot-chocolate mug over as I bounded away. A lake of brown liquid spread over Mickey's dining table.

"Sorry about the table!" I shouted as I slipped past Mickey and disappeared through the door.

Chetna was outside, and we sprinted down Starfish Crescent as fast as we would run a race. The tarmac became sand beneath our feet, and then we were scrambling up the sand dunes, grabbing wet fistfuls of sand and grass to help us climb quicker.

"Get back here!" Mickey was behind us now, struggling to chase us in his mismatched flip-flops. With him now were two security men, dressed in black uniforms with reflective strips on their jackets. "We only want to help you!"

The security guards sprinted after us, their two torch beams reaching through the darkness.

"Keep going, Solo!" Chetna cried. She had almost reached the top of the dune.

I was about to catch up with her when the sand crumbled away beneath my feet. I dug my nails and feet into the wet sand but it was no use. I slid almost halfway back down the dune, spluttering sand from my mouth.

"There!" one of the guards shouted.

My vision went white as their torchlight found me.

I turned and scrambled again, my fingers cupping the sand and my feet digging in. I was climbing, but not quickly enough. Each step I took became two steps back.

"Solo, grab this!"

Chetna launched a frayed and stringy fishing net down from the top of the dune, and a scattering of sand came along with it. The grains covered me, sticking in my hair and eyes. The guards yelled and started spitting sand from their mouths and shielding their eyes. I gritted my teeth and felt the crunch of sand between them. As fast as I could, I hooked my fingers through the holes in the netting.

"Hold on, Solo," Chetna shouted. "I'm going to pull you up!"

Chetna heaved, and I felt myself rising up the side of the dune. Each heave brought me higher and higher, until I could roll myself up on to the top of the dune next to Chetna's feet.

"Thanks, Chetna," I wheezed, getting to my knees. "You saved me. You're surprisingly strong, you know."

"I know," she puffed. "Three years of netball goal attack wasn't for nothing. Now come on – we need to get back to the coach before they send out a search party!"

We slid down the other side of the dune, our socks and trousers filling up with sand and debris as we skidded towards the flat beach. The sea was spitting salty spray, and the wind was so loud it sounded like it was groaning in pain.

"Hurry!" Chetna cried, her voice almost drowned out by the wind.

I looked behind me at Sunset Dunes. I guessed we weren't going to find Morag now.

Chetna and I ran as fast as we could.

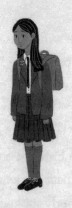

CHAPTER 40

"Come on, Solo!"

My chest was burning, and we were nowhere near the top of the steps that led to the car park. I had counted three hundred and eighty-two slippery stone steps, and there were still more to come.

"I'm trying," I said. My voice sounded weak and weird. I felt sick.

I couldn't stop thinking about Morag. I'd been so sure she would be here. And if she was, we were going home without her. What if she was still here? What if we had checked just one more place?

We got to the final stone step and ran down the alleyway that would spit us out into the car park. The moment we reached the end, Chetna fell to her knees.

"No!" she screamed, her hands on her head. "They're leaving without us!"

"Hello!" I ran across the car park, waving my arms. "Over here!"

The coach was moving off – there was no way they would see us. We watched silently as it slowly took the corner out of the car park and disappeared down the dark street. Nobody looked out of the windows. Nobody saw us.

"Miss Carmichael must have forgotten to do the headcount!" Chetna cried. "Surely she'll notice soon. She *has* to notice. Our names are on the register! Tell me she'll notice, Solo!"

Grimacing, I revealed the scrunched-up class register from my pocket and held it out in front of me. "I might have taken this earlier."

"Solo," Chetna said. "Is that what I think it is? Is that Mrs McDonald's register?"

"I did it so we would have longer to find Morag! Otherwise someone would've realized we were gone."

"But surely Miss Carmichael must have noticed we aren't there?"

"I don't think she noticed us… She was busy when we got on the coach. Mrs McDonald was the only grown-up who saw us, and she's probably forgotten."

All the colour had drained from Chetna's face and her breathing had gone all fast. "I can't *believe* you stole the register. What are we supposed to do now? How are we going to get home?"

"Calm down," I said, thinking fast. "We can always get the train. Me and Morag always take the train when we come here."

"I don't have any money for the train, Solo! I gave you all my money so you could come on this trip!"

"It's fine," I said, starting to feel guilty. "We don't necessarily need money to get the train. It's easy – Morag does it all the time. I promise you, we can get the train back home; and, yes, we might be a *bit* in trouble, but we can blame it all on Miss Carmichael. She should have noticed we were gone!"

"But it's not her fault we—"

"It's all going to be OK, Chetna. I promise."

"*Doors closing.*"

The train doors were already beeping and beginning to creep shut when Chetna and I sprinted on to the platform. We darted along to the very first open door and barrelled through it. We rolled on to the muddy train floor in a mess of limbs and wet clothes.

"Thank goodness," Chetna panted, resting on her elbows. She had a chocolate-bar wrapper stuck to her sleeve. "That was much too close for my liking. Imagine if we had missed it!"

I nodded, but I couldn't speak. My lungs were burning and my heart was hammering louder than I'd ever heard before. I was glad to finally be escaping Normley-on-Sea, even if we hadn't found Morag. The whole place had been nothing but rain, clouds and weird people.

At least we had made it on to the train. Everything was going to be fine. The rain was thudding on the carriage, and the windows were so steamed up we couldn't see outside. All the other passengers were huddled into their jackets or staring at their phones. Nobody even looked at us.

"I simply can't wait to get home," Chetna said, settling into a seat. "I'm going to have a nice hot bath and get into my nice warm bed."

"Same," I said, even though I wasn't sure how warm it would be in the flat. Maybe I would put the heating on. Who cared what Morag would say? It wasn't like she would ever find out. Not now.

A heavy glumness set in. With the palm of my hand, I cleared a circle in the condensation on the window and looked out at the sea. It was the exact same cloudy black as the sky. I could barely see the water, but I knew it was there somewhere, crashing into the rocks and slipping away again and again. A bit like Morag, actually.

A cheerful jingle rang out through the speakers above the carriage doors.

"*This is a customer announcement*," the tinny voice whined. "*Regrettably, this service has been cancelled due to the current inclement weather in the area. We are investigating alternative measures, but this may take some hours. The next train to London departs at 07:49 tomorrow morning. We apologize for any inconvenience caused.*"

A collective groan spread through the carriage.

"No!" Chetna sat upright in her seat. "No! They can't cancel it. We have to get back to London right now!"

I put my head in my hands and closed my eyes. Suddenly I was so tired that I almost didn't care about the train. The doors started beeping again, then they slid open slowly, telling us to get off.

We weren't going back to London that night. Not without a whole lot of trouble, anyway.

*

Outside the train station, Chetna took out her phone.

"We need to call someone, Solo." She pressed the power button, and the screen came to life, emitting a pale light.

"What? No! We just need to find somewhere to sleep. Then we can make our way home first thing tomorrow!"

"And have my parents worrying about me all night? They'll think I've gone missing or something!" Chetna looked like she was about to cry. "My mum won't be able to sleep!"

"You *have* gone missing," I said. "Only we're going home. It's all going to be OK!"

"No, it isn't, Solo!" She was actually crying now; her breath was all jagged and tears were coming out. "We've gone too far this time. How could I be such an idiot, going along with this stupid, *stupid* plan of yours?"

"You're not an idiot," I said. "It was a good plan—"

"You know, I wouldn't have minded learning about coastal erosion and maybe eating a horrible packed lunch on the beach. Too bad that's probably the last school trip I'll ever be allowed to go on."

"I'm sorry, Chetna." I didn't like seeing her upset. I didn't like seeing anyone upset. Why was I always the reason people were upset? "I'm really sorry."

She ignored me and held the phone to her ear. "Dad? It's me."

My heart sank. I could hear multiple voices talking through the speaker.

"I need you to pick me up from Normley-on-Sea. The school bus left without me. I'm sorry, I'll explain later. I know … I know. I'm really sorry. I'll leave my location on so you can find me. OK…"

I walked over to a bus stop and rested my head against the dripping wet panels. So this was how it was all going to end.

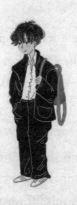

CHAPTER 41

"That's him. That's my dad," Chetna said shakily.

Those were the first words either of us had said in an hour. We had been sitting at opposite ends of the bus stop in a cold, grumpy silence. Chetna was worrying about her parents, and I was worrying about mine, only for completely different reasons. The only sound was the pattering rain.

Chetna got to her feet. A beige car was speeding towards us, flashing its headlights. It splashed through a puddle and skidded to a halt in front of us.

Chetna's dad flung open the driver's door and walked up to her. "What on earth happened to you? Are you OK? How on earth did they manage to leave without you?"

"It's…" Chetna glanced to me, then quickly looked away. "It's my fault, Dad. I wanted to go and buy something from the gift shop. When we finally caught up, they were already leaving."

I stared at the ground. I was grateful Chetna was taking the blame, but at the same time I hated that she had to lie for me again. Perhaps she knew it would give me more time to search for Morag.

"Chetna, that's not like you, not one bit," said her dad. "I'm surprised at you. How could you be so irresponsible? *Anything* could have happened to you! Less than two weeks at your new school and this is how you start acting?"

"I know, Dad," Chetna said, her voice wobbling. "I'm really sorry. I thought we would only be two seconds, and then time ran away from us. Is Mum cross with me?"

"Mum isn't too happy, not happy at all. She hit the roof when she found out they'd left you behind," her dad replied, the steam from his breath billowing in the cold. "But she'll be happier now she knows you're OK. She's at the school talking with Miss Carmichael and the head teacher now. Giving them an earful, no doubt."

"OK." Chetna swallowed. "OK."

"Why are you all wet and covered in sand?"

Chetna just shrugged and stared down at the ground. The silence was awful.

"What was your name again?" Chetna's dad was glaring right at me.

"S-S-Solo," I said. I could barely raise my eyes to look at him. "My name's Solo."

"He's my friend," Chetna said. "It's my fault, not his."

Chetna's dad nodded curtly. "Fine. I'll give you a lift back to school, Solo. They're having a hard time getting hold of your mum, apparently. You'll have to wait there for her to collect you."

A pit of dread opened inside me. Morag wouldn't be collecting me any time soon. "Thanks."

Climbing into the back seat, I wondered what Miss Carmichael and Mrs Howe and Miss Ellis must be saying about me at that very moment. I knew they would be blaming me for making Chetna go missing, and they were right. I was a bad influence. I watched the raindrops trickling down the window, racing out of sight.

We drove back in silence.

It was nearly 7 p.m. when we pulled up in the school car park. Only a handful of cars remained.

There were none of the usual sounds of kids playing

in the playground, or parents arriving for pick-up time. All I heard was the wind whistling and my heart pounding in my chest.

Most of the lights were off at school, except for a few that shone out all yellow like lonely stars. I felt wrong. Like I was in a place I wasn't allowed to be in.

"Come on, you two," Chetna's dad said. "In we go. Let's get this mess sorted out."

Chetna hadn't said a single word in the car. Not that she needed to, because I could already read her thoughts as though I was psychic. A red rash of worry had slowly crept up the skin of her neck and settled on her cheeks. Chetna was scared, and I bet she was starting to wish she hadn't broken every rule in the book just to help Funeral Boy, who she'd only known for a week.

How could you be so stupid, Chetna? she was probably thinking. *Stupid, stupid Solo.*

"I feel a bit sick, Solo." Chetna finally broke the silence as we walked along the path to the main building. Her dad strode ahead.

"It's going to be fine, Chetna. You're new, remember? New kids get away with everything."

"Not this." She shook her head. "Even new kids know not to run away from a school trip and go around a strange town without a responsible chaperone."

Chetna had a point, but I didn't say anything.

"It's my mum I'm worried about. She'll have been waiting for me, getting angrier and angrier." Her voice wobbled uncontrollably. "I've never done anything like this before. I've never really been … *bad*. Until I met you."

The playground was completely empty aside from a huddle of grown-ups at the building's entrance, and a lonely football that rolled around in the wind.

I could make out the shape of Miss Carmichael pacing back and forth. Then a woman with long black hair and colourful clothes. It must have been Chetna's mum. It looked like they were arguing.

Next to them was Mrs Howe. She was talking frantically on the phone to somebody, gesturing furiously with her free hand. Miss Ellis was there too, also on the phone.

"I still can't understand how on earth she just *left* the group without anybody noticing," Chetna's mum was saying. Her voice echoed around the empty playground. "How does something like that even *happen*? Does nobody count the kids? Do you not take a register?"

"I'm sorry," Miss Carmichael pleaded. Her voice sounded strained. She put her palms flat against her forehead as if to cool herself down from a panic.

271

"I promise nothing like this has ever, *ever* happened in my classroom—"

"Or in this school, full stop," Mrs Howe interrupted. "Needless to say we will be conducting a thorough investigation once the dust settles. We are deeply sorry for all the distress—"

"My little girl went missing from your useless school and not one of you noticed. If she hadn't phoned us herself, we'd still be out looking for her. Why, I've half a mind to call the police myself!"

"I assure you," said Mrs Howe, "they have been contacted. And now that we know where Chetna is, we can ensure a thorough and non-biased investigation takes place internally—"

"With all due respect, I will be the one to decide what is necessary when it comes to my daughter being left behind on a school trip, Mrs Howe. Do you understand me?"

Chetna and I heard all this as we got closer, our hearts thumping in unison. I gave her arm a small squeeze. The squeeze was meant to say, *It will be OK.*

I'm not sure Chetna believed me any more though. In fact, I knew she wouldn't want to be my friend after this. Who would? After being forced to skip school *twice*, after getting stranded in a town miles away. I was bad news. The first proper friend I'd made in ages, and I'd gone and blown it.

"I'm here!" Chetna said. Her voice brought silence to the grown-ups. "Mum, I'm here!"

"Chetna!" Everybody seemed to say in unison.

Chetna ran towards the group, her arms outstretched and her shoes slapping on the ground.

"My daughter! Thank goodness you're OK!"

Chetna's mum folded her into one of the biggest, tightest hugs I'd ever seen. I could hear Chetna crying and saying "I'm sorry, I'm sorry, I'm sorry" over and over again.

"Thank God," Miss Carmichael said, tears spilling from her eyes. "Thank *God*." She leaned her head against the wall and let out a massive sigh of relief. I'd never seen a teacher do that before. It was really weird.

The hugs and kisses went on for ages while I just stood there, as though I wasn't really there at all.

"Why on earth did you leave the group, Chetna?" her mum said.

"I told Dad." Chetna was crying again, her breath shuddering. "I wanted to go to the gift shop—"

"Gift shop? *Gift shop?* I don't believe that for one minute, Chetna." Her mum suddenly noticed me and her eyes narrowed. "Did this boy talk you into it?"

Chetna looked at me, her eyes wet and shining bright with tears. "No!"

"You can be honest with us, Chetna," said Mrs Howe. "Solo has a bit of history with this sort of thing. It's important we find out what happened."

Chetna glanced at me, then she let out the biggest sigh ever, like she couldn't hold it in any more. "Tell them, Solo. Tell them the truth. We have to."

All eyes were on me.

"Well?" said Miss Carmichael. "Have you got an explanation for this, Solo?"

I swallowed.

"Truanting is very serious," said Miss Carmichael. "As is influencing another student to do so. There are going to be consequences for this, Solo—"

"No!" Chetna shouted. "It's not what you think. It wasn't like that. You need to listen to him! Tell them the truth, Solo!"

My head felt like a balloon that was about to pop. Everyone was staring at me. If I told the truth, Morag would get in trouble. I would be taken away to the home, just like she'd always said. We'd lose the flat. We'd lose everything.

"Solo, for goodness' sake, just tell them!" Chetna was glaring at me now. Her eyes sent a hundred silent messages. "Or I will!"

"Come on, Solo," said Miss Ellis gently, as she put her phone in her pocket. "You can be honest with us."

I shook my head at Chetna. *Please, no. Please don't do it. Please don't tell. Please, please, please don't tell the truth. Please don't ruin everything—*

"Solo's mum has gone missing!" Chetna blurted out. "He's been living on his own for days. I was helping him look for his mum, that's all. We went looking together, didn't we, Solo?"

"Oh, Solo," Miss Ellis said, coming to stand next to me. "Is this true? You've been on your own? You should have said something, Solo!" She put her hand on my shoulder, which somehow made me feel worse.

"Is this true?" Mrs Howe had gone pale. "How long has she been missing?"

My brain went bright white then. My thoughts went up into the sky like rainwater floating back up to make clouds. I started shaking like my bones wanted to wriggle out of my skin. I tried to shake my head but something, maybe Morag's voice in my head, told me to nod instead.

I nodded yes. *Yes, Morag is missing. Yes, Chetna was helping me look for her. Yes, I've been alone. Yes, yes, yes it's all true.*

I sat down on the cold playground, and it all came flooding out of me. I knew that once I let it all out, it would never ever fit back inside me again, no matter how much I fought and squeezed to keep it down.

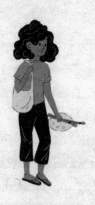

CHAPTER 42

Miss Carmichael was nice to me after I admitted the truth. She kept looking at me and opening her mouth to talk, but then snapping it shut again as if she couldn't find the right words.

She took me inside and let me sit on the comfy chairs in the staffroom. It was weird in there, like another universe. It smelled of old teabags and freshly photocopied paper. The fridge hummed in the background.

Miss Ellis found clothes for me from the spares cupboard. A comfy tracksuit with a hoodie top. "Spares is *not* the same as lost property," she told me. They were brand new, and mine to keep.

I changed into them, then folded up my damp,

sandy uniform and put it in a carrier bag.

Chetna went home with her parents, all three of them arm in arm. I watched them walking out of the school gates from the window. I couldn't decide if I hated Chetna's guts or if I was glad she had spilled the beans. Either way, they weren't her beans to spill. Now my whole life was ruined while hers went back to normal.

Miss Carmichael poured me a glass of orange squash and brought a plate of biscuits and cakes from the teachers' cupboard. Custard creams, bourbons, Jammie Dodgers and a couple of French Fancies. It was a bit like the funeral food I used to have with Morag. I ate the whole lot in one go, and she brought me more. I hadn't realized how hungry I was.

Miss Carmichael kept muttering to herself and sitting down next to me, only to stand back up and start pacing. She did this again and again.

"I'm sorry you never felt you could say something to me, Solo," she finally said. "I had a sense something was wrong, but I didn't want to interfere too much. You wouldn't have been in any trouble at all."

I stared at the patchy carpet. Silence was my best tactic now. Words would only get me into deeper trouble.

"The thought of you sitting all alone at home waiting. It makes me want to…" Her eyes filled up with tears then, and she turned to face the wall. "As a teacher, it breaks my heart, Solo."

I took another custard cream from the plate and washed it down with a gulp of sweet squash.

"Everything's going to be OK, you know," she sniffed. "You'll get through all this mess, one way or another. I should know. I've been there."

"How do you mean?" I said, mumbling through a mouthful.

"My own mum was a bit…" She trailed off. "A bit difficult. She drank too much. Used to go missing and get into trouble. I think that's why I can be rather strict sometimes. It made me prefer rules and routine, rather than chaos and unpredictability."

It was weird. I had never even thought about Miss Carmichael being a kid or even having a mum. I always imagined her hatching as a fully formed teacher from a dinosaur egg in a nest surrounded by fire and twigs.

"I suppose I felt like I was my own mum, really," she added. "You might feel the same sometimes. I felt like I was my sisters' mum too, even though I was only a child myself. It stays with you, that kind of stuff."

"I do cook my own food sometimes. Put myself to bed and stuff. Morag just forgets, that's all," I said quietly.

"I know the feeling, Solo. I really do. You'll learn to find the family you need in many places. I often feel like the kids in my class are my family. If only I'd paid better attention to you, though…"

"Don't be sad about it, Miss," I said. "I'm sure we'll find Morag somewhere. Maybe she'll turn up tomorrow."

She nodded. "I'm sure she will."

"Maybe then, everything can finally go back to normal."

Miss Carmichael smiled sadly. "Maybe even better than normal. It might take some time, maybe years, but you'll realize you're having fun, and you haven't thought about all this trouble in months. That's when you'll know things are getting better."

I couldn't imagine how that would ever happen. All my brain ever did was think about Morag. Where was she? Was she happy? Why is Morag sad? What have I done to upset Morag? I didn't *want* to stop thinking about her, either. The thought of doing that made my stomach twist. Morag was a perfect mum. She was just a bit different.

"For what it's worth, Solo –" Miss Carmichael cleared her throat, then dabbed around her eyes with a tissue that she produced from her cardigan sleeve – "I'm sorry I didn't do more to help. I shouldn't have nagged you about your uniform. It's all so foolish of me, looking back. I feel like a total witch."

"That's OK," I said. "I guess I'll have to give my new uniform back."

She batted the idea away. "It's not important, Solo. We'll sort it. There's more to life than school uniform."

Now *that* was something I never thought Miss Carmichael would say.

"Do you know I call you Miss Cowmichael behind your back?" I asked. I winced after the words escaped my mouth. "I won't call you that any more, though."

She laughed. "Probably a rather apt name, from your point of view. I've heard worse. Hopefully, I can convince you otherwise, in time."

Miss Carmichael extended a hand towards me. I took hold of it, my hand protruding from my hoodie sleeve. We shook hands like proper grown-ups. I think it made her happy. It made me feel a bit happier too.

A distant door slammed and footsteps came clattering down the corridor.

"Where is he?" a man's voice said. He sounded panicked. "Where's my boy?"

"He's just through here," said Mrs Howe. She sounded like she was out of breath. "In the staffroom. That's it – just over there on the right."

The door burst open and a man strode into the silence. He had brown hair with blonde dyed bits at the top, and he wore a black leather jacket. He looked at me, unable to say a word. I couldn't tell if he was happy, sad or something in between.

"Dad?" I shifted on my seat. "What are *you* doing here?"

"Solo," he finally said, panting and heaving. "Thank goodness."

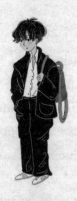

CHAPTER 43

Dad asked twenty-nine million questions as he drove me away from the school. The questions kept coming and coming and I had no idea if they were ever going to stop.

"How are you?"

"Are you hungry?"

"Do you have *any* idea where your mum could be?"

"Any idea at all?"

"How long exactly has she been gone?"

And: "Are you *really* sure you're OK?"

I barely had time to open my mouth before the next question came. They came firing at me like spitballs from Kai Bailey's straw. All I wanted was to think and be quiet. I would have rather been alone in the flat without Morag than sitting in the back of the car dodging Dad's questions.

Eventually the questions stopped and he started talking to himself instead, muttering low under his breath: "I can't believe this!" and "I should've known!" and "I should've done something!" and "How could I be so stupid?"

It was only when he almost drove straight through a red light that he snapped out of it.

There was still a bright red flush on his face and neck. I couldn't tell if he was angry with me or not. Maybe he was angry at Morag. Or maybe he was angry at himself. All I knew was that everybody seemed to get a red flush on their neck when they were with me. Something about me made them feel all weird, and the colour of their neck was the only way they could show it.

Nothing felt right. I didn't like being in the car, and all the swerving was making me feel sick. My stomach was full of cakes and biscuits, and the smell of the jelly-bean air freshener that dangled from the mirror was making things worse.

Street lights and cars flashed by as we travelled through unfamiliar streets. I had no idea where we were going, only that I wasn't going towards home.

After what felt like ages, Dad was driving through peaceful streets I'd never seen before. The houses were all separate rather than stuck together like our flats, and each one had its own garden.

This was what Morag would have called *fancy-schmancy*. She would have done her special whistle that she did whenever something was expensive or posh.

There was a tiny part of me that liked the idea of this new different world, with its mowed front gardens and cars and pet dogs. The hours I'd spent dreaming of a different life – maybe I'd somehow made it all come true. Maybe I should have been more careful with my wishes, because now Morag was gone.

"You can stay with us as long as you want, you know, Solo," Dad said, his eyes meeting mine in the rear-view mirror. "Imelda won't mind one bit. I've told her you're coming. She's been looking forward to meeting you anyway…"

"But I don't want to stay with you," I said.

Dad sighed.

I turned and stared out of the window. I did not want to meet Evil Imelda.

"Nearly home now," Dad said, fingers tapping on the steering wheel to music that wasn't playing. "Won't be long at all."

Evil Imelda was waiting in the doorway when we arrived. She was wringing her hands together and breathing deeply as though she was nervous or something. She looked just like she did in the pictures I'd seen on Morag's phone. Blonde curly hair that stopped before her shoulders, tanned skin without any bags under her eyes. Worst of all, that wide smile that was coated in red lipstick like a clown.

She wore baggy blue dungarees over a stripy top, and sparkly sequinned trainers that Morag would have hated. I almost laughed out loud at the thought of Morag wearing them.

Dad got out of the car, and Imelda ran over and planted a lipsticky kiss on his cheek. Then she leaned into the car and said, "Hello, sweetie pie – you must be Solo. I've heard *so* much about you!"

I faced the other way. I wasn't giving her anything. In fact, I made a silent promise not to speak to Evil Imelda at all. Not one word. It's what Morag would want me to do.

"My name's Imelda," she said slowly, as if she thought I might only speak another language instead of English. "I'm so excited you'll be moving in with us!"

Dad coughed.

"Sorry," she said, looking flustered. "*Staying here* with us for a while. Listen, Solo, why don't you come in? I've made dinner. It's a vegan-sausage casserole with quinoa salad. Do you know *quinoa*? Have you had that before, Solo?"

Dad put his hand over his face and let out a long sigh. A silent message travelled between the two of them, which Imelda seemed to quickly understand.

"What do you say we order a pizza instead?" Dad said. "I can't be dealing with grain salad after the day I've had. I'm sure Solo feels the same."

"I could eat a pizza!" Imelda grinned. "If there's one thing about me, I can always make room for pizza! Do *you* like pizza, Solo? You can have any toppings you like!"

I didn't know why Evil Imelda was talking to me as if I was some sort of baby. Did she not realize I'd been living all alone, caring for myself, searching for Morag, all the while keeping the whole thing secret from every grown-up on the planet?

"Why don't you come on in, Solo?" Dad said. "I'm freezing half to death out here."

I got out of the car and looked up at the house. It was bigger than our flat. Not like a mansion, but it had two floors and its own front door. Warm orange light shone out through the windows and, although I wanted to hate the house, I had to admit it looked quite cosy. It was definitely different from home, where the lights were often off and it was usually freezing, and water was always dripping down the windows.

"This is our home," Dad said, putting his hands on his hips and following my gaze. "Our humble abode, as we call it. It's not much, but it does the job. You can have the back bedroom while you're here. I'll have to move all my guitars and junk out. We'll get the airbed out for you after we've had our pizza."

"I think I'll go for a *white* pizza," Imelda chipped in. "The one with no tomato sauce on the base. It's a bit different but still tasty! Have you had *white* pizza before, Solo?"

I just shrugged. White pizza? I didn't know what she was talking about.

"I need to go upstairs and make some phone calls, love," Dad said to Imelda. "Can you take care of the pizza? Order him something normal, for heaven's sake. Nothing artisanal."

Imelda winked at Dad and squeezed him on the shoulder.

I stuffed my hands into my pockets and followed Dad and Imelda inside. My feet crunched on the gravel path, and it made me think of the funeral that started all this. The one where we walked down the long gravel driveway in the rain and the posh cars drove past us, the passengers staring at us like freaks. Nothing was ever the same after that funeral.

"I heard you've had quite the day in Normley-on-Sea," Imelda said. "It must've been cold. Make yourself comfy while I order."

I stared at the carpet and didn't reply. It was beige.

Homesickness kicked in as Dad slammed the front door and twisted the key with a *clunk*. The door that closed on everything that had happened before. The door that shut Morag out for ever. From the moment that door closed, I knew nothing would ever be the same again. For a second I pictured Morag stuck outside in the cold, banging on the door but nobody could hear her. I shook my head like a wet dog to get rid of the thought.

"Hi there." Imelda was talking on the phone. "I'd like to place an order for delivery if possible? Yep. OK, so it's three small pizzas."

"Large!" Dad shouted from upstairs. "Three *large* pizzas. The boy must be absolutely starving!"

Maybe it wouldn't all *be bad here*, I thought.

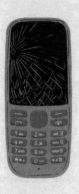

CHAPTER 44

Dad and Imelda's airbed was weirdly comfortable. I slept deeply and for hours. It was a heavy sleep without dreams, with no bloodthirsty packs of TV presenters chasing me, no visions of Morag sleeping rough. I was so tired I probably could have slept on a piece of A4 paper and still found it comfortable.

The next morning, I lay in bed and stared at the ceiling. The plaster had all these white swirly patterns in it like thick meringue. If I looked hard enough, there were faces and shapes hiding in the patterns. I spotted a dog, a tree and a swirl that looked like a snail. But still no sign of Morag.

Someone knocked on the bedroom door. I didn't have my own door in the flat, so it felt quite weird saying, "Come in," as though I was in some sort of office.

"Morning, Solo," Dad said. He was wearing a fluffy pink dressing gown that I hoped belonged to Imelda. "How did you sleep? I hope that old airbed didn't go flat in the night. I must have had it since the nineties. Proper family heirloom, that."

I nodded. "It was all right."

"Good, good." Dad looked awkward, like he didn't know what to say to me. "So, er... What do you normally have for breakfast?"

I shrugged.

"Will toast do? We haven't had a chance to go to the supermarket yet so we don't have much in."

I shrugged again. Buttery toast would do just fine, but he'd have to read my mind to figure that one out. Even better if they had chocolate spread.

Dad looked at the clothes that Miss Carmichael had given me. They were draped over the neck of an electric guitar in the corner. "So, um, we'll take you to get some clothes later on. You'll need something proper to wear. I've got some old T-shirts and stuff you can have for now. You're probably just glad not to be wearing your uniform anyway!"

If only he knew, I thought. The trouble *that* uniform had caused.

I came down for breakfast wearing a pair of red football shorts and a massive T-shirt that Dad lent me. The shirt had a picture of a weird-looking zombie with extra arms and legs on it, and it said **IRON MAIDEN** across the top in huge red letters. I didn't have a clue what that meant. It dangled around my knees like some sort of dress.

"*Yeahhhh*," Dad said when I walked in. "Rock on, Solo. You look like your old pa back in the good old days."

"Oh, Jason!" Evil Imelda tutted. "Why did you have to give him that manky old T-shirt?"

"Well, it was either that or a nice frilly blouse from your side of the wardrobe, love. I'm sure he wouldn't have preferred that!"

"Don't let him wind you up, Solo," Imelda said, rolling her eyes. "You probably listen to *decent* music, like me. Not all that old-man, Dad-rock rubbish."

"Sacrilege!" Dad cried.

I had no idea what either of them were talking about. Dad put two slices of toast with jam and a cup of milky tea on the table in front of me.

"Wait a second – are kids allowed to drink tea?"

Dad asked. "It's not poisonous to them or anything is it?"

"You are so ridiculous sometimes, Jase," Imelda said. "You're not going to poison him. Plus, everyone loves a good cuppa. I'll have one too. Oat milk please."

"Is there any news about Morag?" I asked, chewing the corner of my toast. It was weird hearing my own voice. I hadn't spoken in ages. "Has she come back yet?"

Dad and Imelda shot bizarre looks across the room at each other. They seemed to do that a lot.

"Nothing yet," Dad said. "I've reported her as missing. People are out looking for her. You'll be the first to know when she turns up."

I took out Morag's phone and placed it on the table. There were no new messages or calls.

"They'll probably need to take a look at that," Dad said. Then he took the phone and placed it in the drawer. I wanted to protest, but I didn't. Things suddenly felt quite serious.

"We've spoken to your school as well. You don't need to go back until you're ready. Everybody agrees it would be best."

"Why? Am I being excluded?" That only happened to really naughty kids, and I didn't think I'd been *that* bad. Then again, maybe I had.

"No, not at all." Dad sat down opposite me. "You're not in any trouble. We just think you deserve a break from everything. We've heard things have been tough lately, and people haven't necessarily been very *kind* to you about it all."

"Yeah, to say the least," Imelda cut in. "Those social-media trolls, sitting behind their keyboards. They turn my stomach. We felt terrible when we found out. To think of us swanning around on holiday. Meanwhile, you—"

Dad shot her a look. "Let's pretend none of it's happening. Ignore the whole wide world for a bit."

His words caught my attention. "But Morag's out there somewhere in the world. I don't want to ignore her. I should go looking for her again. There's loads of places I haven't checked yet."

Imelda did a sad smile thing where her lips pursed together. Dad did it too. I was getting pretty used to that strange sad smile. I had a weird feeling nobody was going to let me look for Morag again.

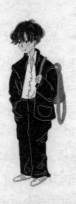

CHAPTER 45

Dad took time off from his job at the council offices to look after me, which I hated. Before, I hadn't seen him in five years; now, I couldn't go five minutes without him asking me annoying questions.

There was nothing to do except wait, so he sat around staring at me while I stared at the wall. Each second felt like it was moving extra slowly, maybe even moving backwards.

Every few minutes, Dad would ask if I needed anything. I would say no because I didn't. Then he would ask me if I wanted a drink, and then go ahead and list every possible drink in the universe: cola, lemonade, cherryade, Lucozade, orange squash, summer fruits squash, apple juice, orange juice, cranberry juice. Oh, and water.

I would say no again, and Dad would ask if I was sure.

Usually I'd get up and walk to another room. Dad would follow me and say, "Well, how about something to eat? We've got toast, cereal bars, cereal, crisps, carrot sticks, pitta bread, apples, oranges, pears…"

Imelda would normally chip in then, and ask if I had ever tried kombucha or fennel tea or something like that. Then she would tell me what it was like being vegan. It didn't sound great, and I didn't want to talk anyway.

On day two of sitting around awkwardly, a police officer knocked on the front door. I saw the fluorescent uniform through the frosted glass and ran to hide in the back bedroom.

I thought they were here about the stolen school uniform. Maybe the shopkeeper from Meagre and Jones had gone to the police after all. When the officer and Dad came into the room, I started telling her how sorry I was. She didn't know what I was talking about, which was a relief. Her name was PC Dolan, and she had come to talk to me about Morag. She was actually pretty nice and smiley for a police officer. I think she was Irish.

Dad and Imelda sat next to me, listening, while

I told PC Dolan everything I knew. I told her about the Big Bad Reds and about the incident at Martin Winner's funeral. I kind of rambled a bit because it was all so confusing and impossible, like untangling a set of earphones. She wrote all the details down in her notebook, scribbling away. Her handwriting was scratchy like mine.

I handed over the note Morag had left behind, which was now so soft it felt like tissue. Everyone looked at each other weirdly when they read it, and Dad started rubbing my shoulder.

PC Dolan said we had to choose a photo of Morag for the police to use in their appeal, on posters and stuff. I scrolled through Morag's phone while everyone watched. There were loads of photos of me, which made a lump swell up in my throat. I chose the photo of Morag and me sticking our heads through the painted board in Normley-on-Sea, the one where she had the body of an octopus. PC Dolan said it was a lovely photograph, but it would be better if Morag looked more like herself, rather than an octopus. I guessed that made sense. Dad helped me choose the photograph of Morag in the red phone box. He said it showed her real personality, which I wasn't too sure about either.

I had to give Morag's phone to PC Dolan even

though I wanted to keep it. She said there might be clues on there, and they would let me know if Morag called it. It was weird not having the phone in my pocket. I'd got used to the weight of it, like a stone that reminded me of Morag.

PC Dolan said I'd done all the right things, and that I'd been "incredibly brave indeed". That was strange. I didn't feel brave and I felt like I'd done everything wrong.

She told me I shouldn't go out looking for Morag on my own again. "Leave it to the professionals," she said. Before she left, she gave us a card with her phone number and email address on it, in case we thought of anything else.

Dad and Imelda ordered Indian takeaway that night to take our minds off it all, but I didn't think it would be so simple. While we waited for the food to be delivered, I sat on the airbed and heard PC Dolan's questions echoing in my brain. *Why did Morag crash funerals? When did she start doing it? Did Morag enjoy it? Were things really that bad?* Anger started to rise like boiling pasta water.

I came downstairs to find curry, naan bread and all the sides laid out across the living-room table like Morag's feast nights. Dad patted an empty space on the sofa, but I sat on the carpet instead.

"Dig in," he said. "Grab yourself a plate. There's plenty of samosas."

For the first time in ages my appetite had disappeared. How could I eat a takeaway with the very person who had caused Morag to go missing in the first place? I put a forkful of food into my mouth and chewed without enjoying it. Dad was chewing too, and suddenly it was all I could hear. *Chomp, chomp, chomp.*

We watched an old documentary about a rock band until finally Imelda got her way. Then we watched a show about people in America trying on different wedding dresses in a shop and arguing about which one to choose with their families. Everyone cried at the end.

"What a nightmare!" Imelda said to Dad. "Mother-in-laws can be the absolute worst, can't they? I hope that doesn't happen at our wedding!"

The wedding. I'd forgotten about the wedding. How could anyone be thinking about wedding dresses when Morag was missing *somewhere* and we had no idea when she would come home? I let half an onion bhaji fall from my mouth and on to my plate. Dad gave me a weird look.

"Something the matter, Solo?" he said. "Try and eat something."

I shrugged and shovelled a forkful of rice into my mouth. I couldn't help but chew more aggressively than usual, even though I knew it was immature. Each angry chew was meant to let Dad know how I felt. He didn't seem to be reading my mind though. He kept eating and laughing at the telly, while my hands started to shake.

A charity advert about homeless people came on during the break. It showed the homeless people sleeping on cardboard boxes, wrapped in sleeping bags and grubby hats and scarves. "*Spare a little love for missing and homeless people this winter,*" it said. "*Donate just five pounds to save a life.*"

Dad and Imelda sprang into action and quickly changed the channel, acting like they were planning to change it anyway. All I could think about was Morag. Was Morag homeless? Was Morag huddled in an old sleeping bag somewhere? It was the last straw.

I didn't notice it happening, but my anger boiled over and escaped my head and now it was out in the real world. I got to my feet and launched my plate of curry hard at the living-room wall. Then I started storming around the place, knocking over a plant pot, punching the stupid scatter cushions on the sofa. I hated everything here.

Dad tried to hold me down but I kicked and punched and screamed and scratched. I wasn't even me – I was an animal smashing its way out of a hunter's trap. It felt good and bad at the same time. I didn't think I was ever going to stop smashing. I didn't ever *want* to stop smashing.

People say that rage is red, but I think rage is actually a cloudy see-through. I could still see everything, hear everything and feel everything I was doing. But I also wasn't there at all. It was like I was watching myself through a dodgy TV screen with the volume off.

"Count to ten," Dad said through gritted teeth, trying to hold me still in one spot. "Try to count to ten, Solo."

"Shut up! Why should I listen to *you*?"

Dad and Imelda looked at each other and somehow had a silent conversation. Imelda rose to her feet and stood across the room, holding a cushion to her chest like a shield.

Dad kept hold of me. "Breathe, Solo. It's OK to have big feelings—"

"I don't *want* to breathe! Why do you even care about me anyway?" I threw myself on to the floor and started clawing at the rug until clumps of it started coming loose between my fingers. Dad pulled me back to my feet and tried to hold my arms still.

"Because I'm your dad! Of course I care!"

"Do you? Because all you seem to want to do is eat stupid curry and talk about your wedding, while Morag's *still missing*. And you know what? It's ALL YOUR FAULT!"

"My fault?" Dad let go, red in the face. "What do you mean, my fault?"

"Because it all started with you!"

I stormed across the room and swept my arm through the display of photo frames on the window sill. There wasn't a single photo of me or Morag there. Only Dad and Imelda getting engaged on holiday. Dad and Imelda horse riding. Dad and Imelda jet-skiing. It almost felt good to hear the glass break as the frames tumbled to the floor.

"Wh-what on earth do you mean?" stammered Dad.

"Do you really not know?" I turned to face him. My eyes felt like they were bulging out of my skull. "If *you* hadn't abandoned Morag and me, Morag would never have got the Big Bad Reds, she never would have lost her job, and we never would have had to go to all those funerals! Then she never would have got in trouble, never would have gone missing, and I wouldn't have to live here with YOU!"

I'd never been in a fight in my life, but saying those things out loud felt like I'd landed a punch.

Red blotches started appearing on Dad's neck and his eyes went all shiny. He looked as if he was going to say something but couldn't choose the right words. Instead, he just shook his head and said nothing.

"Boys," Imelda said. Her voice sounded small and strange. "That's enough now, don't you think?"

It was like a spell had been broken. I was teleported back into myself, standing in the messed-up living room. Bright orange curry was streaked down the flowery wallpaper. Glass crunched under my foot. I bent down and picked up the framed photo of Dad and Imelda's engagement, the one Morag had shown me on her phone. A huge crack had splintered the glass, right between Dad and Imelda's smiling faces.

"I'm sorry," I rasped. "I'm really, really sorry. I didn't mean—"

"Not to worry!" Imelda smiled, but it was the fakest smile ever, like she was clenching her jaw tight to stop herself screaming. "We can replace the frame, can't we, Jason? It doesn't matter."

I looked at Dad, but he wouldn't even meet my eye. He was just staring at the floor, shaking his head to himself like he couldn't believe it. Without a word, I left the room and traipsed upstairs, slamming the bedroom door behind me.

I was turning into Morag. Morag who wasn't even there.

Thanks a bunch, Morag, I thought, not that she could hear me. She'd gone and left me with the Big Bad Reds to deal with. Or the Big Bad See-throughs, in my case.

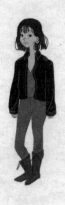

CHAPTER 46

The next morning I woke to find Dad sitting on the end of the airbed. It squeaked under the weight of him like a family of mice. I hadn't slept well. I couldn't stop thinking about the night before. Guilt was churning around in my stomach, making me feel sick. I kept replaying the sound of my plate hitting the wall. The feel of the cracked photo frame in my hands. Dad and Imelda had stayed up for hours, whispering to each other.

"How are you feeling, buddy?" Dad said. "Did you manage to get some rest?"

"Yeah," I croaked, even though I hadn't. "I'm really sorry about—"

"It doesn't matter, Solo," Dad interrupted. "It doesn't matter at all."

"I honestly didn't mean to—"

"We know." Dad patted my legs. "We totally get it. You've been through a lot. More than most people have by your age anyway. It's only to be expected that things get too much sometimes. I'm four times your age, and things get too much for me too."

I lay still. I wanted Dad to tell me off. I deserved to be told off, grounded, banned from watching telly for seven years. That was the only way I was ever going to make up for the damage I'd done.

"Are you not annoyed at me, then?" I asked.

Dad shook his head and smiled. "Nah. Life's too short to be annoyed. Plus, it didn't take too long to tidy things up."

"What about Imelda?"

Dad shrugged. "She gets it. Plus, she'll enjoy shopping for new picture frames. She loves stuff like that."

"OK," I said. I nodded, even though I still felt gross.

"The press have picked up on your mum being missing, buddy."

I rolled over and faced the wall.

"It's probably a good thing, if you think about it.

It might help people to recognize Morag. People will have their eyes peeled for her. Somebody might see her and bring her home."

He showed me the *Daily News* website on his laptop.

FUNERAL MUM MISSING: HAVE YOU SEEN THIS WOMAN? Jack Morley has the exclusive story for the Daily News.

The *Daily News* can exclusively report that viral London funeral-crasher Morag Walker has gone missing, just over a week after she was caught crashing the funeral of celebrity striker Martin Winner.

A source has confirmed that Morag has gone missing previously, and may be in a vulnerable state of mind. Her ten-year-old son (known online as Funeral Boy) is currently staying with relatives.

Morag has been registered as a missing person. Members of the public are advised to report any sightings at the earliest opportunity...

A picture of Morag popped up halfway through the article. It wasn't the picture from the funeral. No snotty Solo in the corner. It was the picture of

Morag that I had taken in London, posing in the red phone box outside the Natural History Museum. She looked happy.

I still hated Jack Morley for hounding us so much, but the article could have been much worse. There were no horrible pictures and no mean headline poking fun at Morag. I crossed my fingers extra tight, hoping the article would help.

Things were weird downstairs, but everyone was pretending to be normal. The living room was tidy, and most of the curry stain had come off the wall. Imelda had gone out shopping, and Dad kept looking at me as if I was about to explode.

That afternoon, Dad got up from the sofa suddenly and slapped his thighs with both hands. He did that when he was going to announce something important.

"Right," he said. "We can't sit around in silence the whole time. Solo, have you ever played the guitar?"

I rolled my eyes. "No, obviously. I can't play any musical instruments."

"Today's the day that changes, buddy. Come on, then, let's go upstairs."

"I don't want to." I sighed. I was tired of his random

suggestions. "I don't care about playing the guitar. I'll only be rubbish at it."

"Well, that's no attitude to have, is it? Come on, you'll never know if you don't try! You could be a future Yngwie Malmsteen!"

"Who?"

Dad rolled his eyes. "Honestly, your generation's ignorance of popular music astounds me. Come on, let's give it a go!"

"Nope. I'm rubbish at everything. Coding, long division, English, PE. I don't want to do the guitar and that's that."

"So you're telling me that a young man who has cooked, cleaned and lived alone at the age of ten, survived going viral *and* initiated a search for a missing person can't even pluck a few strings? I think you're selling yourself short."

I sighed and turned the telly off. "Fine!"

Upstairs in the back bedroom, Dad told me to hold out both arms, then slung a strapped acoustic guitar over my shoulder. I didn't move, just kept my arms in that awkward position, like a shop dummy, not knowing if I was allowed to touch the guitar or not.

"Hmm." Dad bit his lip. "Might be a tad on the large

side for you, but I think we can make it work." He rummaged through the desk drawers and produced something that looked like a metal clamp.

"What's that?" I stepped back, stumbling into the airbed.

"Whoa, whoa, whoa, buddy." Dad helped me back up. The airbed groaned and heaved. "It's for the guitar – I'm not going to clamp your left ear off or anything. This is called a capo; it basically shortens the length of the strings. That should make it easier for shorter arms to reach the bottom fret. Of course, it will skew the pitch upwards a little, but nothing we can do, really. Not until your arms lengthen by a good couple of inches or so."

"What?" I said. Dad was speaking total nonsense again.

In fact, I'd started to wonder whether Dad and Imelda spoke English at all. They had so many words that Morag and I never used. *Quinoa, kombucha, vegan, nuptials, mortgage, Japanese knotweed, kefir, harissa, gut microbiome* and now *capo*. I hardly ever knew what they were going on about.

Dad strapped another guitar over his shoulder and played a few notes. His fingers moved all the way up and down the neck like they were dancing. The sound filled the room and ended with a loud crunch.

I blinked in a daze.

"That'll be you in no time at all," he said, grinning at me. "Well, not *no time*, per se. It actually takes years of consistent practice, dedication and study to become truly fluent with the fretboard. But we can definitely get you playing a few simple chords."

I didn't like the sound of *practice, dedication and study*. It sounded way too much like school, and I was trying not to think about school at all. I was meant to be having a *rest*. Luckily, school didn't seem to be thinking about me either, since nobody had been in touch.

"Perch down here on this chair." Dad directed me to the swivel chair in the corner and sat me down. "Arms like this…"

He arranged my arms as if I was some sort of action figure. One reaching over the fat part of the guitar, the other stretched down the long thin bit. Next, he knelt down in front of me, his tongue sticking out of his mouth in concentration. Then he arranged my fingers into the achiest position ever, like a claw. Then he told me to press down on the strings.

"Hold them down. Now strum across the strings with your other hand."

I pulled my finger across the strings from top to

bottom. It sounded horrible. Most of the strings just went *clunk, clunk, clunk* in a slightly higher sequence of notes.

"Wahey!" Dad started clapping. "Brian May, eat your heart out! There you go, Solo, you've played a C. Your first-ever chord! A momentous moment for any young guitarist. How does it feel?"

I shook the weird feeling out of my left hand. I wasn't sure how it felt. But I noticed I hadn't thought about Morag or trashing the living room in at least five minutes.

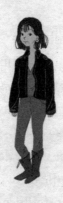

CHAPTER 47

A couple of days trickled by, and we all got sick of sitting around indoors doing nothing, so I started going out to work with Evil Imelda. Annoyingly, I also began to wonder if she was actually that evil. She worked as a professional dog walker, and how could a professional dog walker be evil?

Imelda's company was called Pooches with Paws, which I thought was kind of stupid because didn't all pooches have paws? Maybe that was the whole point. She drove all around the neighbourhood in a special painted van, decorated with bright paw prints and cartoon pictures of every type of dog you can imagine.

On our walks I started to think that being a dog walker was the coolest job in the world. Getting to spend all day with different sorts of dogs, walking around and playing fetch. It sounded better than *commodities*, or whatever Kingsley did. Imelda told me it was harder than it looked, but she couldn't see herself doing anything else.

I got to know some of the dogs. The best ones were a licky brown hound called Monty, a fluffy poodle called Charlie, and a multicoloured dog called Jed. Imelda said Jed was a Heinz 57 because he had that many types of beans in him. I didn't know what she was on about.

Some of the dogs were a bit mean, like those small yappy ones that looked like bony roast chickens with all the meat taken off. Imelda kept those ones away from me and told me what not to do. Don't stare into their eyes, don't make sudden movements, don't make loud noises. It reminded me of what not to do around Morag whenever the Big Bad Reds were particularly big, bad and red.

Usually we took the dogs to the park, but sometimes we drove out of town to an old quarry where the dogs could run around and be crazy. Somehow I always got caked in mud, so Imelda took me to get wellies from the shops. They made a fart sound whenever I walked, which was kind of funny.

"Jason does feel bad, you know," Imelda said one day out of the blue, as we both stepped over a fallen log at the quarry. The dogs were darting around us in the bushes and play-fighting over sticks. "Your dad, I mean. He feels guilty."

"For what?" I asked.

"Everything. For not being around to support you and Morag for so long, I guess."

Morag always told me Dad didn't want to know us, that he was focusing on his new life with Evil Imelda. But he had been teaching me guitar and forcing me to listen to his old CDs. He asked plenty of questions about my life. So I reckoned he did want to know me after all.

Imelda sighed. "He always wanted the whole two-kids-and-a-wife thing, but he just couldn't make it work. Or not with Morag, at least. They both were living a bit of a rock-and-roll lifestyle when they met. But that kind of thing just doesn't last for ever. They fell out of love. I think that was a blow to his self-esteem."

We had talked about self-esteem in PSHE at school. Miss Carmichael told us that *self-esteem* was basically what we thought about ourselves in our heads. She said it was our beliefs and opinions about

315

ourselves, and that self-esteem was important.

"Did his self-esteem go lower?" I asked.

"I think so, yeah." Imelda seemed thoughtful. "He wanted to make everything work. For you and Morag. Things got difficult with Morag after a while, and she wasn't happy. I think they weren't a good match, which happens. It's nobody's fault, of course; sometimes things just don't work out."

"Maybe Morag had the Big Bad Reds all the time," I muttered. "She can be proper hard work sometimes."

"It was both of them, by the sounds of it. Of course, he's never been great at talking about feelings."

I knew what Imelda meant. I didn't like talking about my feelings either. Most of my feelings were bad, or embarrassing, or got me into trouble. Talking about my feelings made bad things happen. It was best for me to press my feelings down, like overstuffing a suitcase.

"He did try to get in touch with you, you know," Imelda said. "He did try to be a part of your life."

"What?" I felt winded. "But Morag said he never… Morag told me he didn't want to…" I stopped, worried I'd say something wrong.

"Yeah." She nodded sadly. "He wanted to look after you every other weekend. Offered to send money. He did send money sometimes in the post, along with your birthday cards and gig invites. Morag said she didn't need it. She sent the cash straight back to him in the exact same envelope. She said she could cope perfectly fine without your dad interfering."

"Dad sent me birthday cards?" I felt all light-headed, as though I might float away in the breeze. I'd never had a birthday card from Dad in my life. "But Morag never gave them to me!"

"I know." Imelda sighed, rummaging through her pockets for dog treats. "I think Morag prefers to cope all on her own. She sent a pretty clear message about that. Then your dad gave up trying to send money and cards."

I couldn't believe what Imelda was telling me. Why would Morag return Dad's money when money was something we didn't have enough of? If she'd taken the money to begin with, none of this would have happened. No funeral crashing, no stealing school uniforms, no baggy suits from the charity shop.

Why would Morag hide away my birthday cards? For years I'd thought that Dad didn't care about me at all. If I ever asked about him, Morag wafted him away like a bad smell.

Anger started bubbling up inside me. Morag never

made much sense to begin with, but every time I learned something new about her, she got even more confusing.

"Don't blame her, Solo." Imelda broke my silence. "She was really struggling, evidently. Plus, everyone gets wound up and overwhelmed sometimes. Morag isn't the only one. Not by a long shot."

"Do you ever get overwhelmed?"

Imelda laughed. "Oh, yes, if only you knew. Sometimes I want to flip my lid when your dad leaves beard trimmings all over the bathroom sink. That's not even the half of it! The Big Bad Reds are actually pretty normal, Solo."

I felt bad again. If Imelda got overwhelmed by a few beard hairs, she must have hated me for throwing a whole plate of curry at the wall. I stared down at my muddy wellies.

We walked on in silence for a bit while the dogs zigged and zagged around us. No one had ever told me the Big Bad Reds were normal. Was it really true that *everybody* got them? I thought Morag was the only one, like she was patient zero and everyone else caught them from her. It felt good knowing that I was wrong about that. Then I felt bad for blaming Morag the whole time.

There still hadn't been any news about Morag. The story had gone into even more newspapers and been on the telly. Dad and Imelda said I wasn't allowed to watch the news, and I wasn't allowed on social media. At first I kicked off a bit, but it was probably a good idea.

"What was Dad's band called?" I asked, changing the subject. Dad talked about his band all the time, but went cagey whenever I asked him about the name.

Imelda smirked. "You honestly don't want to know. Trust me, Solo."

"Go on!" I pleaded. "Tell me. You can't keep it secret for ever. I'll find out one way or another!"

"Fine. They went by the name of the Loco Parentals. Dead cringe, isn't it? They changed the name after they all became dads."

I made a mental note to search for them on the internet when we got home. I didn't know what Loco Parentals meant, but I actually liked the sound of it. I wondered what other history there was to find out about Dad.

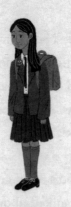

CHAPTER 48

The next weekend, Imelda called me downstairs for breakfast, and there was Chetna standing awkwardly in the hallway with her mum and dad.

"We thought it would be nice for you to have a friend to visit," Imelda said, smiling her big red smile. "Maybe it'll take your mind off things for a bit?"

"Hi, Solo," Chetna said. She shifted uncomfortably. "How have you been?"

"Fine," I said, looking at the floor. "How are you?" I still hadn't made up my mind about whether I was annoyed with Chetna for spilling the beans about Morag when I had specifically asked her not to. "I haven't seen you in ages."

"I know," she said. "I wasn't sure if you were annoyed

with me for telling. I'm really sorry about everything."

"You don't need to say sorry." Suddenly I realized it was true – she didn't need to be sorry. "It doesn't matter. It couldn't go on for ever. You did the right thing."

Chetna's mum walked over and wrapped me in a tight hug. I hadn't expected that a single bit. I held my breath while she squeezed me.

"I felt terrible after that evening, Solo," she said, releasing me. "I wanted to get in touch and tell you that I know it wasn't your fault. We were in shock, and it had been such a terrible day with Chetna going missing from the school trip."

Chetna's dad shook my hand. He wore a chunky silver watch that glistened. "Chetna says you were a good friend to her when she was new in your class. So we want to say thank you for that."

"That's OK," I said. Even though they were saying good things, it was embarrassing. If my head swelled up any more, I would take off like a helium birthday balloon.

"We brought you these," Chetna said, handing me a bulging carrier bag that looked like it was stuffed full of paper.

"Is that all my homework?" I said, my smile dropping.

"No, silly. It's a load of cards from everyone in Miss Carmichael's class. To say sorry about…" She trailed off. "Well, everything, I suppose. Mrs Howe came down pretty hard on Kai Bailey and the Cool Table when she found out how they'd been treating you. Miss Carmichael must have told her. They've been in lunchtime detention ever since, and they feel really bad about it all. We had to have a special assembly about kindness and everything."

"Whoa." I stared into the plastic bag. I couldn't believe that everyone had to have a special assembly because of me.

"Would you two be interested in a cuppa?" Imelda asked Chetna's parents. "You and Chetna can go upstairs and play, if you like. Jason's PS4 is plugged in, in the bedroom. No zombie games though – they're strictly for over-eighteens."

"A cuppa sounds absolutely lovely," said Chetna's mum. "I'm parched."

"Wonderful," Imelda said, clapping her hands. "I've baked a vegan Victoria sponge too, if I can interest you in a slice or two?"

"I'm meant to be avoiding sugar," Chetna's dad joked. "But you've gone to all this trouble. I suppose you can count me in for a slice…"

Upstairs Chetna and I got all the cards out and spread them across my airbed. They were all handmade out of A4 crafting card folded in half. Everyone had used the full range of colours, and some people had even stuck sequins and stickers on the front.

Hope Your OK, the first card said. It was written in big green bubble writing, and the colouring was neat and within the lines.

Thinking About You, said another. This one was covered in multicoloured felt bobbles and pipe cleaners.

I picked up one card that had scratchy handwriting and a shaky drawing of a thumbs up on the front. *I'm Sorry, Solo*, it said on the front. It was from Kai Bailey. *Sorry about the egg chucking and being horrible. I won't be horrible to u any more. Do u want to play footy with us lot when u get back? Let me no what u think. Kai B.*

We Miss You, Solo! another card read. *Very much looking forward to having you back in class. Don't worry about schoolwork in the meantime. Mrs Howe has sorted the uniform thing with the shop. Everything will be OK. All the very best, Miss Cowmichael.* She had stuck a laughing-crying emoji sticker and a cow sticker next to that. Miss Carmichael's card made me laugh.

Thinking of you! said the next one. *Dear Solo – thinking of you while you're away. I am always here for a chat if you need anything or even if you don't! From Miss Ellis.*

"This one's from me," Chetna said. She picked out her card. On the front she had drawn neat little sketches of things we'd done together: a pair of scissors, a drawing of a squirrel, a mobile phone, a smoothie in a glass, a boy and a girl running across some sand dunes.

Thanks for being a great friend, it said. And inside: *Let's be friends for ever. Everyone is thinking of you loads and loads. I'm coming over to your dad's house to play tomorrow, but it's a surprise. Well, I guess you know now because you are reading this card LOL. Love from Chetna.*

Chetna helped me place the cards around the room so I could see them all. They took up the whole of the desk, the top of the chest of drawers and the shelf above the airbed. It was almost like I was getting a card back for every birthday card that Morag had stashed away. But I knew I shouldn't be *too* happy or smile too much. Morag was still out there, somewhere, and I wanted her back.

I showed Chetna the chords I'd learned on Dad's

guitar: C, G, D, and E minor. The notes sounded rubbish and tinny, but Dad said that was enough to start learning some easy songs for beginners. He told me he'd ordered a half-size guitar for me off the internet, so I could reach the fretboard better. It would arrive soon, and we could start our own band just like the Loco Parentals.

Imelda would be on lead vocals, I would play rhythm guitar, and Dad would play the lead. All we needed was a drummer, then we could be just like Pixies, according to Dad. Maybe it was Fairies, I'm not really sure. Chetna told me she was starting the clarinet next term, so maybe she could join the band too. That sounded pretty cool, actually.

Afterwards, we went downstairs and ate huge slices of Imelda's cake with everyone else. It was weird being with so many people at once. Everyone was chatting and it was hard to know when it was my turn to talk. I stayed pretty quiet and let Chetna do the talking for me, which I didn't mind. She told everyone how good my guitar chords were, and everyone looked proper pleased, especially Dad.

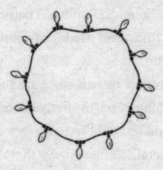

CHAPTER 49

A few days later, Dad and Imelda took me back to the flat to pick up some of my things.

The unopened pile of post for Morag had only grown bigger: more bills, more letters about rent. Our laundry was still hanging on the radiator in the hallway. It was like time had stopped ticking while I'd been gone. Dad bundled the dry clothes under his arm and brought them inside.

My heart was hammering when we pushed the front door open. Even though Dad and Imelda told me not to get my hopes up, I had still expected Morag to be there when we arrived, sitting at the kitchen table waiting for me. Instead all we found was silence and the dim, dusty kitchen.

"I'm sorry, buddy," Dad said, patting me on the back. "I know you were hoping she'd be here. I think we were too."

"It's OK." My lip sort of wobbled, but I bit on it with my two front teeth to stop it. "I knew she probably wouldn't be, deep down."

I was determined to be brave that day, but being back in the flat without Morag made it too real. I had sort of been pretending I was on holiday while I'd been staying with Dad and Imelda. But no Morag meant the holiday might have to become my normal life, and I'd have to say goodbye to my old life for ever. I pushed that thought away. Morag was coming back.

"I'll tell you one thing," said Dad. "It's a while since I've been in this flat. Must be about five years. I barely recognize the place."

Dad pulled the curtain back and light filled the flat. The rain had mostly washed the egg stains from the window, so now it only looked like bird poo.

"Morag definitely made the place her own after I left, that's for sure." He ran his finger along all the fairy lights that were stuck on the walls. "She always loved these."

"Is this where you used to sleep, Solo?" Imelda asked. She was peering behind the sofa into my alcove.

I'd forgotten nobody was supposed to know about my corner, but it was too late now. She'd seen it.

"Most of the time," I said. "Or in Morag's bed with her. I prefer my corner though – it's really comfy. Usually Morag chats to me over the back of the sofa and tells me stories."

Imelda seemed sad for some reason. "We're going bed shopping on the way home, Jase," she said to Dad. It wasn't a request. "He's not sleeping on that manky old airbed any more. He needs a proper bed."

I didn't see the point in going bed shopping. I'd only be sleeping in it for a few more nights, and then Morag would be home, and everything would be back to normal. It seemed like a giant waste of money to me, but sometimes Dad and Imelda liked to waste their money.

I'd noticed that they didn't always have the supermarket versions of things that came in the white-and-red packets. Things like custard-cream biscuits and honey-nut cereal. When we went food shopping, they would choose the more expensive ones in nice boxes with pictures on the front and free toys inside.

One time, Imelda told me I could pick one treat from the food shop, so I chose one of the mini pizzas from the fridge bit. I loved the way they tasted. The doughy base, the tangy tomato sauce, the stringy yellow cheese on top. They were only 65p, and they were my favourite. Imelda put it back on the shelf and swapped it with a rectangle-shaped sourdough pizza that had long bits of salami and something called artichoke hearts scattered on top. The artichoke hearts tasted bitter. I picked them all off and put them in the bin when no one was looking.

I started walking around the flat and picking up my things. I closed up my throat really tight so no feelings would escape. I got my toothbrush from the bathroom, my blanket from my alcove. I fished my pyjamas out from the laundry pile and stuffed them into my backpack. I stashed some toy cars that I hadn't played with in years, and an overdue library book from under my pillow.

Next, I found my crumpled funeral suit by the bed where I'd left it. I knew I would never wear the suit again, but I wanted to keep it anyway. Memories were stitched inside the fabric like threads. Memories of Morag rolling up my sleeves again and again, tucking in my shirt when it came untucked.

In my corner, I grabbed the photograph of Morag and me from our holiday in Normley-on-Sea, the one where we stuck our heads through the holes, and I was a diver and Morag was an octopus. I wondered if I would ever go back to Sunset Dunes again.

"Is that everything?" Dad asked. "You can take whatever you like, you know."

I scanned the flat. Flecks of dust were swirling around in the sunlight. I wanted to take *everything* with me, the whole flat. The sofa, the telly, the kitchen table, Morag's bed, the alarm clock, the bathtub, the wooden chairs, my mattress, the fairy lights. I would have taken Morag's toothbrush with me if I could, but she would need that when she got back.

"Just one more thing," I said.

I stepped into the bathroom and unhooked Morag's fluffy polka-dot dressing gown from the back of the door. It was too big to fit in my bag, so I slung it over my shoulder. She would want this when she came home, and I would be the one to give it to her.

"Are you ready to go, Solo?" Imelda put her hand on my shoulder and rubbed it. "We can stay a bit longer if you want."

"No." My voice sounded really dry and weird. I coughed to clear my throat. "I think I'm ready."

Dad locked the front door behind us, and I had a horrible feeling that I wouldn't ever be coming back.

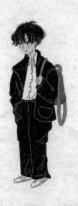

CHAPTER 50

Dad and Imelda had three small arguments while they were building my bed. They weren't proper fights so it was actually kind of funny. Watching them pretend-arguing took my mind off Morag and the flat.

Dad tried to build the bed without reading the instructions first. Imelda said he always did that, and that's why it always went wrong whenever Dad built anything. When it then went wrong, Imelda said, "I told you so," and Dad got proper huffy about it and started sweating everywhere.

It was a really cool bed, so it was worth it. Dad told me it was called a *loft* bed, so that's why building it was such a "pain in his proverbial", whatever that was.

The bed was raised up high off the floor, so there was space for drawers and a desk underneath, as well as a hidey corner for me to get cosy. Lying in bed, I could touch the swirly meringue ceiling with my hand. Each morning, I slid down the ladder like a kid in an American film.

I wondered what Morag would say when she saw the bed. She probably would have done that whistle when she thought something was proper fancy. I kept Morag's polka-dot dressing gown upstairs and used it as a blanket.

Dad and Imelda's spare room slowly started turning into my room. Dad and Imelda bought me a blue duvet set, cushions and LED strip lights to go round the ceiling. The half-size guitar Dad bought me online arrived, along with a stand, a rainbow-design strap and a book of guitar chords for me to practise. Most of them were too hard because, no matter how much I tried, I still only had five fingers on each hand.

Chetna came over again with her parents the next weekend. This time, she brought me eight books from the school library. Apparently, Mr Mohammed, the school librarian, said I could keep them as long as I wanted, and not to worry about the return date. There was a book about Egyptians, one about crystals that grow underground, but my favourite was a giant book of world records and wackiest facts. My favourite world record was the longest fingernails ever. The fingernails snaked out of the woman's hand like elongated pork scratchings, which was both gross and cool at the same time.

This time, we all went out together to a place called Old MacDonald's Country Park, which was super cool. It had rides and slides, and animals you could actually touch. I held a baby piglet with ginger hair. The lady in charge of the animals said the piglet liked me. Morag would have loved the piglet. Some of the rides were a bit babyish, but we went on them anyway because it was funny.

The day after, Imelda took me to get my shaggy hair cut at her favourite hairdresser's called Balayage. The hairdresser offered me a hot cup of herbal tea and a head massage before they started trimming, which was weird. The tea smelled amazing, but actually tasted like watery mud, and I spat the tea out all over the cloak. Imelda got embarrassed but said it didn't matter. She gave the hairdresser an extra ten-pound note to say sorry about the tea-spitting thing.

The routine in Dad and Imelda's house started to feel kind of normal. Every morning, Dad got up first, showered, then loudly brushed his teeth, which always woke me up. For breakfast I had toast or cereal and a cup of tea, and we always listened to the radio while we ate it. Dad and Imelda would get annoyed at the politicians being interviewed, but I never knew what they were talking about anyway.

I carried on going to work in Imelda's van, and I got to know all the dogs. Imelda lent me a special dog-walking lead that went around my waist like a belt, so I could walk five dogs at a time. She gave me the older and best-behaved dogs to walk so they wouldn't trip me up and drag me away down the street, never to be seen again.

I was still off school "having a rest" while everything got sorted. Not that I would admit it, but part of me was starting to miss it. Not the work, obviously. But Chetna, and Miss Ellis, and the smell of lunch wafting from the canteen. Being stuck at home made the days feel endless.

Staying busy was the only way I could keep Morag at the back of my mind. Whenever I didn't have anything to do, Morag would come crashing back into my head, and I would feel guilty, then start worrying again. One thing I learned is that I was very good at worrying about Morag. It was one of my talents.

PC Dolan kept in touch with Dad about Morag's case. Dad wouldn't tell me the details, no matter how much I bugged him. He let slip that Morag had supposedly been spotted walking around central London. Another time, someone thought they saw Morag sitting alone in the back row of a funeral service at Southwark Cathedral. By the time they went over, she had gone.

Hearing this made me feel strange. I started to wonder if Morag could be right under our noses, walking around London, sneaking down alleyways, crossing roads. I kept my eyes peeled whenever we left the house, scanning the streets for a woman in black with a lacy black hat hiding her eyes.

One day Imelda stopped her van at a junction to allow a funeral procession to pass. My heart clenched up inside my chest. Neither of us spoke as the cars slowly rolled by. There was no sign of Morag.

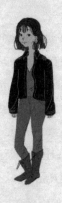

CHAPTER 51

I was there when the call finally came. I knew it must have been important because it came through on Dad and Imelda's home phone, which never rang at all. The noise it made was shocking, like it was dividing the past and the future with its horrible high-pitched ring.

"Jason speaking," Dad said, sounding cheerful. But his face dropped, and he started scrabbling around for a pen and a piece of paper. "Crikey, yes, speaking," he said, flustered. "Correct."

"*Is it her?*" Imelda whispered, as she handed him an old receipt and an eyeliner from her handbag to use as a pencil.

Dad batted her away, and she came and sat next to me and squeezed both my hands. I tried to squeeze back, but mine were shaking. I had wanted to know so much what had happened to Morag, then suddenly I didn't want to know at all. I wanted everything to stay the same. Not knowing anything was much better than knowing something bad for certain. Wasn't it?

Imelda turned down the volume on the telly so Dad could hear properly. Dizzy, I watched the newsreader's lips moving without any sound coming out.

"Right," Dad said. His voice was catching in his throat. "Right, I see."

"Solo," Imelda whispered, "whatever happens, we're here for you. OK, sweetheart?"

"That sounds like her. It sounds a lot like her, yes," Dad said. "Is she talking? Where was she found?"

"Thank you," I whispered to Imelda.

"Right," Dad said. "Thank you for the call. Thank you for letting me know." He placed the phone in its holder and wiped his forehead with the back of his hand. He looked pale and shaky suddenly, not like him at all.

"What's happened, Jase?" Imelda stood up from the sofa. "Is it her? Has she been found?"

"Solo," he said, eyes glistening and red. "It looks like we need to make a trip to the hospital."

"Right now?" I said. Suddenly I'd forgotten how

to move. My whole body felt numb, as if it had been switched off at the plug and only my brain was awake. "Is she OK?"

"She's a little worse for wear." He nodded solemnly. "Are you ready?"

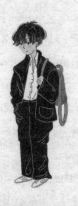

CHAPTER 52

I never liked the smell of hospitals. They smell like cleaning and chemicals and medicine and the inside of the first-aid kits at school. All those smells remind me of bad things happening. People falling over. People getting cuts and bruises. People breaking their arms and legs and catching flesh-eating diseases. People having operations and having to swallow horrible bitter pills. People dying.

Dread swilled around in my stomach as Dad and I searched for someone to ask for directions. The hospital had even more corridors than school. There were so many people. Doctors and nurses rushing about, pushing beds through double doors and taking hurried notes on clipboards.

Sounds of phones ringing and bleepers bleeping and people talking and alarms ringing everywhere pressed inwards on my eardrums like fingers. I jogged to keep up with Dad's mega-fast strides, but I wasn't tired because I knew – I *hoped* – we were finally about to see Morag.

When we found the right ward, the woman at the ward reception desk took a million hours to look up from her computer screen. Dad was getting impatient and kept rolling his eyes and shifting his weight from one of his suede boots to the other. Eventually he cleared his throat loudly and the receptionist stared at him, as though she was annoyed we were there.

"Name?" she said, not even bothering to say hello.

"Uh." Dad fumbled and stuttered like he'd forgotten how to talk. "My name's Jason Walker. This here is my son, Solo Walker."

The woman rolled her eyes and huffed out a big sigh. "Not *your* name. I need the patient's name. Who exactly are you hoping to visit today?"

"Oh, I'm sorry. We're here for Morag. Morag Walker. I believe she's recently been brought in. She's been, er, missing for around three and a half weeks. Are you a nurse?"

"I am." The woman raised her eyebrows, in the way

that people always seemed to do whenever Morag was mentioned. "I know the one you mean. Head down this hall here, then take a right, then right again. You'll find her in the private room at the end of the corridor."

Dad looked to me blankly, then back at the nurse.

"Is she OK?" he asked. "How has she been? Is there anything at all you can tell us? She's been missing, you see. We're at a total loss here."

The nurse swivelled in her chair to pick up a brown folder stuffed with loose pieces of paper. She flicked through the sheets until she found what she needed to know. Her eyes danced across the words without expression.

This was it, the moment I'd been waiting for. I crossed my fingers tightly inside my pockets, then crossed my toes inside my shoes.

She tossed the brown file to one side and shrugged. "She'll live. You'll see when you get in there. She's sedated but well. We've managed to settle the tremors down for the most part. The doctor will be able to tell you more."

"Tremors?" I asked, looking to Dad. "What are tremors?" They sounded like some kind of bug that lives inside your stomach. Dad just shook his head like, *How on earth should I know?*

"Is she awake?" he asked.

The nurse shrugged again. "To an extent. She's drowsy, worn out. They've calmed her down a lot. She was shouting about funerals when she came in."

"What about the Big Bad Reds?" I asked, finally plucking up the courage to speak. "Is she all better now?"

She smiled at me blankly, as though I was speaking a foreign language. "I'm not a hundred per cent sure what you mean, sweetheart. But you're in luck – it's visiting hours, as it happens."

"Brilliant," Dad said. "Can you tell me…"

He and the nurse kept talking, but their voices faded into muffled background nonsense. Nothing else mattered any more. Morag was here, and she was *alive*. Alive enough to be awake and talking, even if it was about funerals still. *My* Morag.

Relief started to rise from me like the steam from a pot of instant noodles. It rose into the air, higher than me, right up to the ceiling. My eyes started leaking out of the corners and I blinked hard. *Morag was alive.*

"Come on then, Sol. Let's go and find her."

Dad set off walking and I sprinted beside him. Every next corridor felt longer than the one that led to it, stretching out for miles. I wanted to run ahead and burst through each and every door until I found the one Morag was waiting behind.

All to the left and right were beds full of poorly people, some connected to wires and contraptions, others watching antiques on the telly and dozing off. Some looked so old they were like skeletons. A couple of people had yellow skin the colour of a fading bruise. One patient had a stomach that was as round as a beach ball. Another was stick-thin like the caveman remains I'd seen at the Natural History Museum. I tried not to stare.

Would Morag look like a skeleton, or would she be the same as when she'd left? Would she still have the same eyes and smile? I wondered whether she would be connected to wires and tubes and machines like a computer receiving an update.

Then a question popped up, a bad question. A question that I tried to loosen from my head like a wet dog shaking off rainwater. *Would Morag even be happy to see me?*

Dad stopped outside the final door. It was labelled ROOM 204. He looked pale and worried, like he was trying to hold his trembles inside his body. I knew exactly how he felt.

"Are you ready?" he said. He bent down so his eyes

were at the same height as mine. "It's OK if you want to wait a minute. Or if you want me to go in first – that's absolutely fine too. It might be difficult, whatever we find in there."

"I'm ready," I said. I could barely keep my hands still. I reached past Dad and pulled the door handle down. "I want to go in *now*."

"You sure?"

"Surely sure."

I pushed open the heavy door to the private room, and there she was. Morag. Or the rough shape of her at least, mostly covered by bed sheets. She was lying with her back to us, her messy black hair sprawled out across a plump white pillow.

Above her head, a small whiteboard was stuck to the wall. On it, some scratchy handwriting said: *Call me Morag. Don't mention funerals.*

My body felt electric with anticipation. I held my breath as I took in the slow rise and fall of her shoulders. We listened to the slow puff of her breathing and the sound of it catching in her throat, like a tiny cough. We watched as she started to turn herself over in bed. First she arranged her elbows, then the rest of her followed.

Morag looked tired and thinner than she usually did. Her skin was a pale shade of yellow. I could see the bones underneath her neck. A plum-coloured bruise stretched from the top of her cheek and all the way down to her mouth. It looked sore.

There were plastic tubes going into both her arms, and bandages were wrapped around her hands and elbows. Bits of dark, dried blood were seeping through. The sight of it made me feel queasy. I swallowed down hard.

Morag stared at me and Dad, her eyes roaming slowly across the two of us. Her face was blank, like she'd never even seen us before in her life. It was as if there was not a single thought going around her brain.

She'd forgotten all about me. My eyes started burning and a huge lump started growing in my throat.

But then Morag smiled.

"Solo," she whispered. Her voice was all quiet and croaky. "Solo, my lovely boy."

"Morag!"

I ran over to the bed and pressed my weight against her body, careful not to get caught up in the tangle of wires and tubes that hung around her like a spider's web. I buried my face into her shoulder and felt her skin and bones and hair and inhaled the smell of her.

It was really her, it was Morag, and she was alive, she was here. Everything was going to be OK.

Tears started coming out of my eyes and this time I didn't even try to stop them. My shoulders were shaking. I didn't know whether I felt happy or sad. I felt a mixture of every feeling I could name, along with millions more that I couldn't.

"Where did you go, Morag?" I eventually managed to say. My voice sounded strange, all thick and gloopy with tears. "Where did you go? I was looking everywhere!"

I felt Morag's tears dripping down too, splashing like fat raindrops on the top of my head. She pulled me even closer, into the tightest hug I've ever had.

"Oh, you know. Here and there," she croaked. "Got out of town for a bit. Passed through Normley, actually. Thought a bit of sea air might lift me up. It wasn't the same without you, though."

"Normley?" I *knew* I had been right to search there. I must have been too late. "I *looked* for you in Normley!"

Morag shook her head. "I'm sorry, love. You wouldn't have wanted to find me anyway. I was in a bit of a state, to be honest." She ruffled my hair. "You've had your hair cut. Nice and smart."

"I don't care about my haircut!" I cried. I knew I sounded babyish. "I was worried about you!"

"I'm really sorry, Solo," she said. "I never meant to scare you. I've really let you down this time, I know I have. It's not good enough. I'm so, so sorry, love."

I squeezed her even harder. "That's OK, Morag."

"No, it's not. I'm a mess. It's not good enough for you, me being like this. You deserve better. You deserve the best."

"But I don't want better!" I cried. "You are the best! And you're here now. Everything can go back to how it was."

"It can't, love," she whispered. "It can't go back to how it was."

"Why not? Why can't things go back to normal?"

"Because it never *was* normal, Solo. I've been a mess. I haven't been very well up here." She tapped her head with her finger. "That funeral business got into my brain, I think. It's addictive, in a way. And even though I love you so, so much, it isn't fair for you to have to put up with all that at your age. You should be having *fun*."

I nodded, even though it hurt inside my chest. "The Big Bad Reds."

"Yeah. But I'll promise you one thing, Solo, and

I want you to listen to this. I am going to get better. No matter how long it takes, or what I have to do. I think we've both had enough of this nonsense now, don't you?"

I nodded again, even though I hated what she was saying. That things wouldn't be the same.

"And when I'm better, maybe then everything can get back to normal. Although I've never liked that word much: *normal*. Only boring people are *normal*. We'll be something way cooler than *normal*. It might take a little bit of time, but we'll get there. OK?"

"OK," I said, sniffling.

"You know you're my favourite boy in the whole universe, don't you?" She wiped my tears away. "The only one I'll ever need. That's why I called you—"

"Solo," I whispered, my voice hitching. I wiped my nose on the sleeve of my sweatshirt and left a massive snot stain.

"I'm really sorry, Jason," Morag said, looking at Dad over my shoulder. "To you and Imelda. You've been looking after him, then?"

"It's been our pleasure," Dad said with a little shrug. "Don't even mention it. He's family. So are you, Morag. No matter what's happened between us, all right? None of that matters, not really."

Morag nodded and pulled me in close again. We stayed like that for ages, like stone statues locked into the tightest hug on record. Morag and me. Like always.

After what felt like ages, there was a knock on the door. A nurse in a baggy blue uniform came in, holding a tray of food. It seemed to be a tuna-melt panini, a side of mac and cheese, and a glass of luminous orange squash. Weirdly, I felt hungry after all those big feelings.

"Hello again, Morag," the nurse said. "Oh, this must be your boy, Solo!"

"Yep." Morag smiled. "Isn't he perfect?"

"A fine young specimen!" She grinned. "Every bit as lovely as you said he would be. Pleasure to meet you, Solo. I'm Nurse Winnie. I've been helping to look after your mum."

"She's doing a grand job too," Morag said, winking. "Winnie makes the best cup of tea on the ward, if I do say so myself."

Nurse Winnie batted away Morag's words. "Stop it, you'll make me blush. All part of the job." She set the tray down across Morag's bed. "Now, I hate to say it, but visiting time is coming to an end for today. But we'd be delighted to have you in again tomorrow."

"But we've only just got here!" I said, looking from Morag to Dad. "I don't want to go yet!"

Dad cleared his throat. "What do you say we leave Morag to get some rest, Solo? We can come back tomorrow."

"Your dad's right, Solo," Morag said. "I won't be going anywhere, not in this state. I promise you I'll be right here."

"I'll be keeping my beady eye on her, don't you worry!" Nurse Winnie added, smiling.

"OK," I said. "Tomorrow. In the morning?"

"Brilliant," Morag said. "Maybe you can bring me in one of those celeb mags to keep me entertained?"

"You got it, Morag." I did a feeble double thumbs up. My hands were still shaking a bit. "I'll bring you whatever you need."

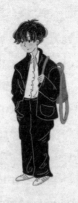

CHAPTER 53

Choosing Morag's daily magazine became a ritual, just like a morning bowl of chocolate cereal. Dad and Imelda would take me to the supermarket, and I spent ages staring at the rack of magazines, dazzled by the colours and photographs of famous people.

The magazines had zingy names like *Hi!* and *Today!* and *Surprise!* even though the stories written inside didn't seem zingy at all. Some of the stories were mean, a bit like the stories that were written about Morag and me. Mostly they were about famous people getting divorced, or getting sick, or getting caught drunk. It seemed weird that Morag wanted to read about strangers having a hard time, when she was going through a hard time herself.

Usually I would take some sort of present in too. I would choose a box of chocolates, gummy sweets, flowers or grapes, luminous bottles of fizzy drink. Soon Morag was so surrounded by flowers and presents that she started sharing them with other patients on the ward.

Dad and Imelda didn't mind, even though the presents must have been costing them a lot. They saw that buying Morag's magazine made me feel like I was helping. I think they were as relieved as I was that Morag was OK.

Well, she was OK-ish.

One morning I arrived and Morag didn't want to talk. Her eyes were red and puffy like she'd been crying. She managed a croaky "Thanks, Solo" when I handed her the magazine and jelly sweets I'd brought. Then she rolled over and closed her eyes. I guessed Morag's low mood hadn't totally gone away.

While Morag slept, I sat in the visitor's chair wondering if I'd done something wrong. Nurse Winnie smiled at me whenever she came in. After a while, she asked if I wanted to help her with her nurse jobs while Morag rested.

Nurse Winnie took me around the ward and showed me what everything was. She showed me the nurses' station, where they did all their paperwork and had cups of builder's tea. She showed me the toilets and a crane-looking machine called a hoist, which they used to lift people into the bath. She even let me stick my head into the sluice room, where they flushed away people's sick. That bit made me feel gross.

The only proper job I did was sorting out the thank-you cards that previous patients had sent in after they'd got better. There were tons of them, all with different pictures and handwriting inside. Nurse Winnie said they got so many cards they had to display them on rotation. I liked the cards. They made me feel that Morag would get better too, just like all those people before. Maybe she would send in her own thank-you card one day.

When Dad came to collect me, Nurse Winnie told him that I'd been very helpful indeed.

"Nice, Solo!" He beamed. "Getting in a bit of early work experience, are you? Perhaps a career in the medical field awaits."

I shrugged. I wasn't sure if flushing away people's sick was the job for me. But I did like the chatting and cups of tea.

"We'll be seeing you tomorrow then, Nurse Solo!" Winnie winked.

"I'll see you tomorrow, Winnie." I gave her two thumbs up.

Other visits went better. Morag and I would play Connect Four on the tray over her bed, even though most of the pieces were missing. I had a feeling Morag was letting me win, because my prizes started mounting up. We only played for chocolates, but I won so many I said I never wanted to eat chocolate again. Obviously, I wasn't being serious.

Sometimes Morag got tired of games, and we would read the magazines in silence. Often I would turn to show Morag something crazy from one of them like "*I put twenty-one Crème Eggs in my mouth – and survived!*" but she had drifted off.

School started sending homework to Dad via email, which I hated. At least it gave me something to do when Morag fell asleep. It was only little things: reading a website about coding, or researching protein. I had a feeling I wouldn't get in trouble if I didn't do the work, but something made me want to show Miss Carmichael I could do it, especially after what she said to me that night.

Morag's skin turned less yellow by the day, and the bruise on the side of her face faded to pale pink, the colour of a blackcurrant-squash stain. The wires were removed from her arms, but she still had to take tablets. Three times a day Nurse Winnie would come in with Morag's pills sorted into little paper cups. Morag would groan, but took them all anyway, swilling them down with water.

Winnie said Morag was very well behaved, which made a change. Maybe everything would be fine after all.

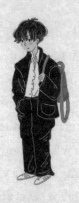

CHAPTER 54

During one visit I was asked to wait in the Family Room on my own while Dad, Morag and the doctors had a private chat. They said the chat was strictly for grown-up ears only. I whined that I wanted to stay, but Dad gave me a raised-eyebrow look that said the decision was made.

I hated the Family Room. Nobody used it, and it smelled like the chemicals the cleaners mopped the floors with at school. There was a broken vending machine, a wobbly coffee table, several mismatched chairs, and a weird roller-coaster toy made of wires with threaded beads to push along. I didn't play with it because it was for babies.

There was a tiny portable telly in the corner, but the

remote control was broken and the picture was flickery and grey. I tried to watch cartoons but quickly gave up. I scuffed the toe of my left shoe into the carpet to pass the time.

I noticed that I could see straight into Morag's room through the thin glass window in the Family Room door. I couldn't help but peer in, trying to read their lips and figure out what was so top secret. Maybe they were talking about me.

Morag was sat up in bed, surrounded by Dad and two doctors. She looked upset. Her face was all crumpled and puffy. She kept dabbing the corners of her eyes with a scrunched-up tissue that looked like it was about to disintegrate.

Dad was perched at the end of Morag's bed. He looked serious. He kept slowly nodding like he was deep in thought, then looking between Morag and the two doctors. Whatever he said made Morag cry even more, but she still nodded in agreement.

My arms and legs felt tingly, as if something bad was happening. Maybe Morag wasn't getting better after all. Maybe she wasn't coming home. Maybe she was dying. My eardrums started pounding.

I pushed my nose up against the glass, but the condensation from my breath clouded my view. I wiped it away with my hoodie sleeve, but then one of the doctors stood in the way of Morag. I only saw snippets of action, like photographs cut up with scissors. Dad reaching out to pat Morag's hand. Morag rolling over in bed. Dad cupping his head in his hands. The doctors walking to the door and going out.

Before the door swung shut, I saw Dad stand up. He ran his hands through his hair and let out a big puff of air. He looked worried. He glanced over at the Family Room door and caught me staring. His eyes and mouth went wide.

I ran to the other side of the room and quickly turned up the volume on the little telly. Some cartoon for babies was on but it sounded like static. I pretended to watch it closely, kicking my legs back and forth. Dad opened the door.

"Hey, buddy," he said, leaning against the door frame. "Enjoying your cartoons?"

"No," I mumbled. "The telly doesn't even work. It's rubbish."

He laughed. "It wasn't exactly a cakewalk in there, either."

"What's a cakewalk?" I asked. "Sounds all right to me."

He shook his head. "It doesn't matter."

"Why was Morag crying?" I asked. "What were you talking about with those doctors?"

Dad sat in a chair with orangey-yellow foam leaking through the seams like chunky sick. He was staring at the floor in the way that people always did when they didn't want to tell me the truth.

"Is it because she's…" I tried to swallow through grit in my throat. "Dying?"

"What?" Dad moved to sit beside me and put his arm round my shoulders. "Is that what you've been thinking?"

I shrugged my shoulders, even though I really meant *yes*.

"Oh, Solo." Dad rubbed my back. "No, Morag isn't *dying*. She's doing really well. She's going to get *better*, Solo."

I felt warm relief spreading all through my body. It felt like my blood had started flowing after being frozen solid inside my veins. I let out a slow breath.

"But what were you talking about?" I said, after a few silent seconds trickled past.

Dad shuffled in his chair. "So here's the thing, Solo. For Morag to really get better, she needs to go away for a little while. For some rest."

"But she's had some rest!"

"It's complicated. You know the Big Bad Reds? That's what you and Morag call it, isn't it?"

I nodded.

"Well, she needs to learn how to live with her condition in a way that doesn't hurt her or you. That's going to be quite the task, and she's going to really need to concentrate on that for a while. If she goes home now, she might not figure out how."

I nodded again.

"The doctors think – and Morag agrees – that it's better for her to go to a special place to get better. Somewhere they'll really know how to look after her and help her manage what she's been going through. Does that make sense? There's a place called Cedar Hall with a bed ready for Morag. They're going to take excellent care of her."

I nodded *again*.

"So this means you're going to be staying with me and Imelda for a while, OK? Maybe a few weeks, maybe a bit longer. We'll have plenty of time for guitar lessons, and you can help Imelda plan the wedding. Chetna can come over whenever you like. We'll make it fun. How does that sound?"

"Fine," I said, picking at some dried chewing gum

that was stuck to the arm of my chair. My eyes were blurry. "When will Morag go to the special place?"

Dad sat back in his chair and let out another sigh. "Today. So why don't we go in now and have a chat before she goes?"

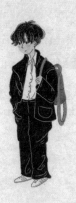

CHAPTER 55

In Morag's room, Nurse Winnie was already gathering Morag's things and placing them into a holdall. Cards, presents, chocolates, clothes. Every trace of Morag was being neatly packed away.

"Hello, my boy," Morag said, sniffing. She looked all crumpled. "I take it you've heard the news?"

"He has. I've told him everything," Dad said, coming in behind me. "Took it like a real trooper as well. He's a tough kid, this one."

"Come here." Morag patted the space next to her on the bed. I climbed on top of the mattress and leaned into her arms. She smelled fresh and clean, like strawberry shower gel.

"How do you feel about it all, Solo?" she asked. "Do

you understand why I've got to go away for a while?"

I nodded, then buried my face into her arm. Tears were fighting their way past my eyelids and I didn't want anyone to see.

"It's OK to be a bit sad," Morag said, rubbing my arm. "It is sad. I'm really going to miss you, Solo. It's been lovely having you visit me here."

"I'm going to miss you too, Morag," I mumbled into her arm.

"But I'll tell you something. I won't be gone for ever. I guarantee it will fly by – ten times quicker than you can even imagine."

I hoped Morag was right. The last few weeks had felt like the longest time ever, especially when Morag was missing.

She carried on. "When I get back, I'll be a whole new person."

I knew Morag was trying to make me feel better, but her saying that made me feel worse. I didn't want a whole new person; I wanted an old one. Morag. The old Morag, just like before.

"Can I still come and see you?" I asked, wiping snot from under my nose.

"I expect so," Morag said quietly. "Once I'm settled in. But I want you to have a rest too. It's no fun spending your time in hospitals at your age. You should be out playing, making messes. Not stuck in here watching me snooze all day."

"But I don't mind," I said. "I really don't mind!"

Morag smiled and messed up my hair. "I know you don't. You're good like that."

"That's everything packed up, Morag." Nurse Winnie emerged from the bathroom with Morag's toiletries in a carrier bag. Her eyes were glistening. "The transport team is waiting, whenever you're ready."

Nurse Winnie walked over to the bed and held Morag's hand for a moment.

"Thanks for everything, Win," Morag said. "You've been amazing. Thank you for keeping Solo busy too."

"Don't mention it, Morag. You focus on getting yourself better. Then you'll be back with Nurse Solo before you know it!"

"I will." Morag squeezed Winnie's hand.

Two men in green uniforms knocked on Morag's door. They said they were going to help move Morag.

Morag exhaled. "Well, I guess this is it, then."

I nodded, biting down on my lip. I couldn't even look at Morag, even though I wanted to soak in every memory of her before she went away.

Morag gave me one last kiss on top of my head.

"Promise you'll be good for Dad and Imelda, yeah? And try not to be too sad. I'll be back home before you know it, Solo."

"I will. I'll miss you, Morag," I said. "I'll write you letters!"

"I'd love that, Solo," she said as the bed began to move away. "I'll miss you!"

She waved as the men manoeuvred the bed out of the door, and then Morag was gone. Me and Dad stood in silence in the empty room. The only trace of her was the whiteboard tacked to the wall. *Call me Morag. Don't mention funerals.*

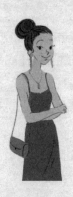

CHAPTER 56

Six months later

I'm still living at Dad and Imelda's house. I quite like it now. Things are definitely different. It's strange how much things can change in so little time.

I like my guitar lessons with Dad. I've learned a few more chords, and the ache in my fingers is going away with practice. Dad gives me his old CDs to listen to, and I want to learn how to play every song. Maybe I could even be in a band like Dad and the Loco Parentals. Dad says I should try to be a "Solo" star, but he's just being cringe.

I go out dog walking with Imelda at the weekends. I love helping out with all the dogs, meeting the new puppies that come along. Imelda reckons I should work with animals when I grow up. So that's two things I'm good at now, apparently.

I feel guilty about calling her "Evil Imelda" before, because she's not evil at all. I told her about it and said sorry. She said I wasn't the first person in the world to believe in the whole evil stepmother thing, and I wouldn't be the last. She said as long as we get along now, that's what's most important. Imelda's pretty cool, actually, and she's better at talking about feelings than Dad. That's OK, because everyone's good at something different. That's what she told me.

School is better too. Chetna and I have lunch together every day, and now that our tables have been rearranged, we sit together too. Goodbye Cool Table, but I guess they're not that bad. Even Kai Bailey is nice to me now. Sometimes he asks if I want to play football. Turns out I hate football, but it's nice to be asked.

I still get sad when I think about Morag. I've found that the easiest way to feel better is to write her a letter and post it to Cedar Hall. She usually writes back in a day or so, telling me what she's been up to. Usually she seems happier. I think she's getting better. It's weird remembering our old life together.

The worst bit is the guilty feeling whenever I

admit that things are easier now. Dad says I should try to focus on the good memories over the bad, but sometimes they make me sad too. *Morag will always be a part of you*, he always tells me.

I still love my loft bed. I like being high up, looking down over everything. Dad printed out loads of photos of Morag and me, and they're all tacked along the side of the bed, so I can look at them whenever I like. The photo of us at Sunset Dunes is still my favourite, even after everything that happened there.

I like the way the bedroom door closes and I can be all on my own with my thoughts if I want to. When I don't want to be on my own any more, all I have to do is leave the door open and Dad and Imelda come in to see me. Sometimes Imelda brings me snacks, which always goes down well.

Today my door is open and there's loads people in the house. I can hear their chatter and laughter downstairs and people keep frantically rushing this way and that. There's a lady here to do Imelda's hair, and another lady doing Imelda's make-up. Some of Dad's mates are downstairs too, dressed in suits and ties and shiny black shoes. They're acting weird and nervous and excited.

I should've said, it's the wedding day. Dad and Imelda will be husband and wife by lunchtime.

My new suit is hanging on the outside of my wardrobe. It's light blue, with a fancy waistcoat and a fresh white shirt to go underneath. The sleeves end just at my wrists, and the trousers just above my feet. No rolling up required. I still have my old funeral suit in my wardrobe. Sometimes I run my fingers over the fabric and the memories come flooding back.

"Hey, buddy!" Dad knocks on the door even though it's open. "Ready for the big day? How did you sleep?"

I scrunch up my face. I was too nervous to sleep much. Whenever I closed my eyes, I pictured myself tripping up as I walked down the aisle and dropping the rings down a drain. I don't know why there would be a drain in the middle of a church, but you never know. I lie and tell Dad I slept fine.

"Good lad, Solo. Well, I've got something special here for you to take care of," Dad says, smiling. Then he produces a tiny brown leather box from his jacket pocket. Inside are the very golden weddings rings I was dreaming about. They shimmer and twinkle in the daylight.

I can't help but stare. This is the first time I've seen them, and they're amazing. Our reflections shine back at us from the gold, our faces shrunken to a tiny version of ourselves.

"I want you to guard these rings with your life, OK?" Dad says. "Then when the vicar asks you to *please present the rings*, you know what to do, right?"

"*Please present the rings*," I mutter, trying to remember my cue perfectly. I act out handing over the box with the rings inside.

"Nailed it!" Dad laughs. "Seems like you know what you're doing. That's when you hand them over to me, OK? Then that's your job done – party time!"

I nod, though secretly I'm worried I'll mess the whole thing up.

Dad ruffles my hair with his hand, making it all stick out in different directions. "I'm proud of you, buddy. I'm so happy you're here with us today. And every day, for that matter."

I go red.

"I'll leave you to get into your suit, Sol. Give me a shout if you need help with your tie, OK? There's no judgement here – I'm well over forty years old and I still struggle to tie my own."

"Will do, Dad."

Before he leaves, he gives me a pointy-finger wink and a big smile. I do it right back at him, even though it's cringe.

"Another thing," he says, lingering by the door. "We've got a big surprise for you today. No guessing, OK?"

"You're not making me play guitar, are you? Because I won't do it, Dad."

"You'll see!" He runs away, laughing mischievously. I roll my eyes.

Outside the church I start to feel sick. The car ride was too bouncy, the bells are ringing too loud, and I can't even hear myself think. Suddenly I'm not sure I can do this.

Imelda is standing behind me in her long, white fairy-tale wedding dress, and all around me are bridesmaids in puffy pink dresses and strange people I've never seen before. The bridesmaids are Imelda's nieces, and they keep looking at me funny.

I feel hot and sticky in my new suit, and a part of me wishes I was wearing my old baggy one instead. I shouldn't have eaten so much breakfast. What if I throw up and ruin the wedding?

A shaky hand starts to rub my shoulder.

"Bit nerve-wracking, isn't it, Solo?" Imelda says, bending down to whisper in my ear. She smells of flowery perfume and powdery make-up. She's trying to make me feel better but her voice sounds trembly and scared. "I feel the same, don't worry. I never actually thought this day was going to come!"

I don't dare reply in case my breakfast reappears when I open my mouth, so I nod and focus on the stone floor, my heart pounding like an orchestra of drums in my chest. Organ music starts to blare out. My stomach somersaults and I plead with it to stay inside me where it belongs.

Imelda squeezes my shoulder even tighter now. "You've got this, Solo. Just like we practised. Pretend that nobody's here."

I give her a smile. She will officially be my stepmum after today. It feels strange but OK at the same time. I like Imelda a lot.

I have a secret, by the way. Imelda and Dad told me they are having a baby. I have a little brother or sister on the way. It's only tiny now, so I won't say anything to anyone. Not yet. Secret-keeping is another thing I'm good at.

I take my first step into the church, right after the bridesmaids. What feels like a thousand people in dresses and suits all turn round and eyeball me. Everyone is smiling. I hear someone whisper that I look cute in my new suit.

My legs become putty as I slowly walk down the aisle, like I'm walking a tightrope in a circus. I press my hand against my chest pocket and feel the box with the rings inside for the thousandth time.

Chetna waves to me from the side, where she's standing with her mum and dad. She's wearing a really cool dress with fabric that wraps over her shoulder and gold stitching. Her mum is wearing one too. The gold-patterned stitching glints in the light. Chetna gives me two thumbs up, and I do them back.

There are more faces I recognize too. Miss Ellis is standing next to Chetna and her family. She gives me a subtle wave and a wink, and I can't help but smile. I still wear the pair of shoes she gave me, even though my toes are creeping towards the ends and the Velcro is coming loose. I think I'll probably keep those shoes for ever, even when my feet are twice the size.

Next to her is Kingsley, buttoned up in a fancy-looking striped suit. He's kept in touch with Dad and Imelda, and I think they're sort of friends now. He came to their barbeque the other week, and he says he'll get me work experience when I'm old enough, so I can have a briefcase kind of job like his. I'm not sure if he's being serious, but we'll see.

Halfway down the aisle my balance goes wonky and I stumble. I stop and turn round, even though at the rehearsal they told me just to keep walking forward, no matter what. Everything feels weird. Up feels like down. My head is dizzy, and my fingertips tingle like they're filled with popping candy.

I look behind me. Imelda is waiting to enter the church. She's lit up by the sun, like an angel in a film or something. She's smiling, her eyes all shiny with tears. She gives me the thumbs up and a little wave, and I feel a bit better.

Then I turn back to face Dad, who is waiting at the front of the church for Imelda, and for me. He's smiling too. He's *beaming*. He beckons me forward, and the wedding guests start to chuckle a bit.

"*You can do it, Solo!*" a voice whispers from somewhere to my side. "*Keep on going!*"

My eyes flick to the side, following the voice, and all my thoughts trickle out of my brain. It's Morag, smiling at me from her seat. She's got tears in her eyes, but she looks happy.

"Surprise, Solo!" she says. "My smart, handsome boy. I love the new suit!"

I blink and blink again. It's really her. It's really Morag. Back from Cedar Hall where she went to get better.

Morag looks so different that I almost don't recognize her. She's wearing this fancy green dress the exact same colour as fresh grass. Her hair is all shiny and neat, and it's tied up in a fancy plait that looks a bit like a Belgian bun. Her skin is no longer yellow and grey – she's healthy and awake, with rounded cheeks and sparkly eyes. Her dark purple bruises have long faded away.

She looks so … *pretty.*

"Morag!" I finally blurt out. I'm still not sure if I'm dreaming. I'm breathless, but my chest still swells up with pride. "You're here!"

"Of course I am, you silly doughnut. I wouldn't miss it for the world! Listen, we'll have a catch-up at the reception afterwards, OK? I've got loads of great stuff to tell you. Now go on, Solo son. Everyone's waiting!"

I glance around me and Morag is right. Everyone in the church is looking at me, smiling, willing me to keep moving forward with a kind light shining out from their eyes.

"You can do it, Solo," she whispers. Morag shoots me a special wink for good luck and I shoot her one right back.

I walk down the aisle, unable to flatten my smile. Everyone is here: Morag, Dad, Imelda, Chetna. And a baby brother or sister on the way. I used to feel like I was all alone, that I was the only one. Solo, just like my name.

But I have a suspicion I won't be solo any more.

ACKNOWLEDGEMENTS

Working in the books world, I know how many sharp minds and capable hands go into shaping every manuscript and the books they become. So, here's my attempt at thanking everyone involved in *The Boy in the Suit* without filling another book entirely with names.

I must first thank my wonderful agent, Chloe Seager at Madeleine Milburn Literary Agency, the first person to truly "get it". Thank you for all you and the team at MMA have done for this book. Equal thanks to Lauren Fortune, a close second place if "getting it" were a race. Your combined input has been truly instrumental.

To Wendy Shakespeare and Genevieve Herr, huge thanks for your keen eyes and help unpicking those tricky narrative knots. Things would be so very tangled without you. Thanks to Sarah Baldwin for the beautiful design, and to Tika and Tata Bobokhidze for the illustrations, which have truly brought the characters to life.

Thank you to everyone in the sales, export, marketing, publicity and production teams at Scholastic. Personal thanks to Emma Kirkby, Ed Newbon, Sjenka Harvey, Chris Ratcliffe, Gordon Knowles, Lucy Page, Tina Mories, Antonia Pelari and Catherine Bell for your support.

Endless thanks to the authenticity readers and experts who so generously gave their time and lived experience to inform how Solo and Morag interacted with the systems and people in their world. This guidance has been beyond helpful, thank you.

I'm lucky to have beautiful friends who have supported this entire process and provided vital distraction when needed. I won't begin a listing exercise, partly due to the fear of missing someone important, and partly because I truly have no idea where to draw the line. To those friends who have listened throughout, expressed support, sent me cat videos to watch, I thank you immensely.

To my family, a paragraph will never suffice, so the whole book is for you. Thank you, Bob, Ria and Dave, for your unimaginable support and all the laughs. To Mum, who would have led the cheer every step of the way, thank you. To my wonderful nephews, Francis, Alastair and Henry, thank you for unwittingly lending me your voices and turns of phrase. Keep on talking – I have another book to write! To Tom Morrison, thank you for being the best foundation and most dependable listener anyone, let alone me, could ask for.

Thank you to the entire Morrison family for your kindness and encouragement.

Finally, I'd like to acknowledge you, the reader. Thank you for clearing the time and space to spend with this story – that truly is half the battle of reading. I hope you have enjoyed a glimpse into another life and were entertained along the way.

FURTHER INFORMATION

If you have been affected by any of the issues in this book, you are not alone, and advice and help is available.

The **Trussell Trust** supports a nationwide network of food banks, working to provide emergency food and support to people facing hardship:
www.trusselltrust.org/what-we-do

If you have been inspired to help food banks support their communities or campaign for change to end the need for food banks in the UK, you can find more information here:
www.trusselltrust.org/get-involved/fundraise

Childline can help with a range of issues affecting children, including anxiety, bullying and family problems. They have a free helpline as well: 0800 1111.
www.childline.org.uk

The **NSPCC** (National Society for the Prevention of Cruelty to Children) provides support with dealing with bullying, and can also support children whose parents are dealing with poor mental health.
www.nspcc.org.uk

Our Time supports children who have a parent with a mental illness, and understand that it can be a difficult and overwhelming experience for young people.
www.ourtime.org.uk

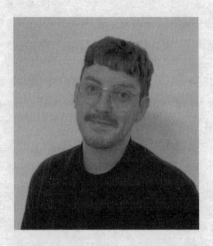

JAMES FOX

James Fox works in children's publishing and previously worked as a children's and YA books buyer for retail. James has picked up writing credits for the *Huffington Post*, *LYRA* magazine, *Door is a Jar* journal and *Flash Fiction Magazine*, and has taken writing courses with the Poetry School and City Lit. *The Boy in the Suit* is his debut novel.

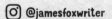 @ScholasticUK 　 @jamesfoxwriter